Current Topics in Microbiology
174 and Immunology

Superantigens

Edited by B. Fleischer and H. O. Sjögren

With 13 Figures

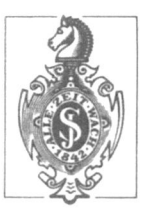

Springer-Verlag
Berlin Heidelberg NewYork
London Paris Tokyo
Hong Kong Barcelona
Budapest

BERNHARD FLEISCHER

Pathophysiology Section
First Department of Medicine
University of Mainz
6500 Mainz, FRG

HANS OLOV SJÖGREN

Wallenberg Laboratory
University of Lund
22007 Lund, Sweden

ISBN 978-3-642-51000-7   ISBN 978-3-642-50998-8 (eBook)
DOI 10.1007/978-3-642-50998-8

© Springer-Verlag Berlin Heidelberg 1991
Softcover reprint of the hardcover 1st edtition 1991
Library of Congress Catalog Card Number 15-12910

Typesetting: Thomson Press (India) Ltd, New Delhi;
Offsetprinting: Saladruck, Berlin; Bookbinding: Lüderitz & Bauer, Berlin.
23/3020-543210—Printed on acid-free paper.

Preface

This volume of *Current Topics in Microbiology and Immunology* is concerned with a class of molecules that are the most potent polyclonal stimulators of T lymphocytes of several species. These molecules have been named "superantigens" because they use a mechanism of T cell stimulation closely mimicking MHC-restricted recognition of specific antigen: they act on variable parts of T cell antigen receptors and are presented by MHC class II molecules.

Prototypes of these molecules are the pyrogenic exotoxins produced by *S. aureus* and *S. pyogenes*, of which the staphylococcal enterotoxins and the toxic shock syndrome toxin are the best known. Superantigens also occur endogenously in mice, most notably the enigmatic Mls determinants, that have withstood characterization for nearly 20 years. Only very recently was it found that *Mls* is probably encoded by endogenous retroviruses. The list of candidates that are implicated as being superantigens is growing. In many cases, however, the proof that a given molecule indeed falls into this category is still missing.

Most of the chapters in this volume are concerned with the effects of superantigens on T cells. Although they cover the same basic issue, they focus on quite different aspects, either on the molecular mechanisms involved or on the biological implications. The overall mechanism of T cell stimulation is the same for the different molecules, and a basic consensus model is generally accepted. Certain features, however, are still controversial, e.g., the requirements for coreceptor molecules or the question of V_β specificity. In addition, individual superantigens differ in several respects, e.g., in receptor specificity or pathophysiological significance.

The extreme potency of these molecules is reflected by a number of biological consequences that contribute to the pathogenesis of the diseases induced by the producing microorganisms. Besides the mitogenicity for T cells, a common feature of all microbial superantigens is their ability to induce shock-like symptoms, probably at least in part due to a massive release of lymphokines and monokines mediated via T cell stimulation. A similar shock syndrome is observed after administration of mitogenic anti-CD3 antibodies to patients for immunosuppressive therapy.

Common to several, perhaps all superantigens is an ability to induce immunosuppression. Several mechanisms can be envisaged as contributing to this effect: most importantly, besides clonal deletion, the induction of clonal anergy in those T cells responding to a given superantigen, the induction of cytotoxicity against MHC class II-positive cells, and the massive polyclonal stimulation of T cells that could impede a coordinate immune response. *M. arthritidis*, a natural pathogen for mice and rats, produces the superantigen MAM and offers a particularly convenient model system to study the role of a superantigen in the diseases induced by an infections pathogen. MAM induces shock and immunosuppression and is likely to have an influence on autoimmunity and the development of a chronic inflammatory disease in the host.

Progress in the field of research on these molecules has been extremely rapid in the last 2 years. In a fast moving field like this it is inevitable that several important developments will have taken place by the time this volume appears in print. A first example of this is the fact that the retroviral origin of *Mls* and related murine superantigens was published after submission of the manuscripts for this book. We can expect further exciting findings in the near future.

B. FLEISCHER, H. O. SJÖGREN

Contents

List of Contributors

(Their names can be found at the beginning of their respective contributions.)

Molecular Genetics of Pyrogenic Exotoxin "Superantigens" of Group A Streptococci and *Staphylococcus aureus*

P. K. Lee and P. M. Schlievert

1 Introduction

Many bacteria require a complex set of host-parasite interactions in order to cause disease. Perhaps the most straightforward of these interactions is elaboration by the microbe of toxins which induce disease manifestations. In this example the pathogen must only be able to survive and multiply within the host for a sufficient period of time to make the toxin. Toxin-host cell receptor interactions then determine the extent of host tissue damage.

Group A streptococci and *Staphylococcus aureus* are extracellular pathogens which make a wide variety of exotoxins and exoenzymes that contribute to their capacity to cause disease. Among these factors are cytotoxins, such as hemolysins, strepto- and staphylokinase, nucleases, proteases, hyaluronidase, and a large family of exotoxins, the pyrogenic toxins. In adition, *S. aureus* makes two serological types of exfoliative toxins, A and B, which share V_B-restricted T cell mitogenicity with the pyrogenic toxins; exfoliative toxins, however, are not pyrogenic and do not predispose the host to lethal endotoxin shock, and thus are only distantly related to the pyrogenic toxin family.

Pyrogenic toxins include the streptococcal pyrogenic exotoxins serotypes A, B, and C (synonyms SPEs, scarlet fever toxins, erythrogenic toxin type A, blastogen A type A, lymphocyte mitogens, and keratinocyte proliferative factor),

Box 196 UMHC, Department of Microbiology, University of Minnesota Medical School, 420 Delaware Street Southeast, Minneapolis, MN 55455, USA

Table 1. Shared biological properties and disease association of pyrogenic toxins from *Staphylococcus aureus* and group A streptococci

1. Pyrogenicity
2. Enhancement of endotoxin shock
3. T lymphocyte mitogenicity; leads to:
   a Enhancement of delayed hypersensitivity
   b B cell immunosuppression
   c Monokine release from macrophages

Staphylococcal enterotoxins also induce vomiting and diarrhea when given orally to monkeys. This property is not shared with the other toxins. Similarly, SPEs are more likely than the other toxins to predispose the host to significant myocardial damage

staphylococcal toxic shock syndrome toxin-1 (TSST-1), staphylococcal enterotoxins (SEs) serotypes, A, B, C1, C2, C3, D, and E, and staphylococcal pyrogenic exotoxins serotypes A and B. These toxins share many biological activities, summarized in Table 1, and are though to play a causative role in several important diseases, including toxic shock syndrome, toxic shock-like syndrome, streptococcal scarlet fever, and staphylococcal food poisoning.

In this review we examine the molecular biological and biochemical relatedness of pyrogenic toxins. Since they can be separated into subfamilies based on sequence similarities and shared epitopes, the toxins are presented according to these subfamilies.

2 Toxic Shock Syndrome Toxin-1

The TSST-1 gene, designated *tst*, was cloned originally into *Escherichia coli* by KREISWIRTH et al. (1983). Chromosomal DNA from *S. aureus* strain RN4256 was partially digested with *Mbo*I, and the 7-10 kilobase (kb) fraction was isolated and ligated to *Bam*HI-digested alkaline phosphatase-treated pBR322. The ligation mixture was transformed into *E. coli* strain 259 (LOFDAHL et al. 1983) with selection for the pBR322 Ap^r marker. Transformants were screened for insertional inactivation of the pBR322 Tc^r marker, and toxin-positive clones were selected by a colony immunoassay using rabbit anti-TSST-1 antisera. A comparison of periplasmic shockates with a lysate prepared from shocked cells indicated that most of the TSST-1 was contained within the periplasm when expressed in *E. coli*.

After *tst* was further localized by subcloning in *E. coli*, the gene was reintroduced into a TSST-1-negative *S. aureus* strain RN4220 (KREISWIRTH et al. 1983) using plasmid pE194 (HORINOUCHI and WEISBLUM 1982). TSST-1 toxins produced in *E. coli* and *S. aureus* clones were identical to the native toxin in physicochemical and immunological assays. The cloned toxins migrated with the same molecular weight under SDS-PAGE analysis and focused at the identical isoelectric point as native toxin. In addition, the cloned toxins were identical to the native toxin in the following biological assays: pyrogenicity, enhancement of susceptibility to lethal endotoxin shock, T lymphocyte mitogenicity, and immunosuppression (KREISWIRTH et al. 1983).

TSST-1 was also introduced into *Bacillus subtilis* by ligating the *tst* gene to *Bacillus* plasmid pBD64 (OKUBO et al. 1972) and transforming into *B. subtilis* IS75. Interestingly, the *B. subtilis* clone expressed fourfold more toxin than the donor staphylococcal strain (KREISWIRTH et al. 1987a). Bacillus-derived toxin, which was released into the culture media, appeared to be identical to native TSST-1 but was less soluble in water.

Nucleotide sequencing of TSST-1 showed that the *tst* structural gene consisted of 702 nucleotides, coding for a protein (Fig. 1) of 234 residues (BLOMSTER-HAUTAMAA et al. 1986b). The first 40 amino acids, representing the signal peptide, were absent from the mature protein as shown by N-terminal sequence analysis of mature TSST-1 (IGARASHI et al. 1984; BLOMSTER-HAUTAMAA et al. 1986b). Thus, the coding sequence of the mature protein was 194 amino acids in length, and the predicted molecular weight was 22 049. This is in good agreement with the previously reported molecular weight of TSST-1 (22 000) as determined by SDS-PAGE (SCHLIEVERT et al. 1981; BLOMSTER-HAUTAMAA et al. 1986a). Computer analysis of the amino acid sequence showed that TSST-1 has little or no sequence similarity with biologically related toxins (SPEs and staphylococcal enterotoxins) (BLOMSTER-HAUTAMAA et al. 1986b). However, a possible significant degree of similarity exists with SPE A and with SEA when computer alignments are used that match conservatively substituted amino acids (BETLEY and MEKALANOS 1988).

In an initial survey of 13 TSS isolates KREISWIRTH et al. (1982) were unable to demonstrate involvement of phage or plasmid in production of TSST-1. They proposed that the *tst* gene is located on a genetic determinant that is capable of heterologous chromosomal insertion and is unlinked to several well-characterized genetic markers. SCHUTZER et al. (1983) later showed that many strains that produce TSST-1 were lysogenized by temperate bacteriophage. These investigators proposed that lysogeny in *S. aureus* may by responsible for pathogenesis of TSS. However, KREISWIRTH et al. (1983) subsequently provided convincing evidence that lysogeny was not involved in TSST-1 production. They also showed that lysogenic phages from toxigenic *S. aureus* strains do not carry *tst*.

The TSST-1 genetic element is absent in nontoxigenic *S. aureus* strains (KREISWIRTH et al. 1983). There appears to be multiple but a limited number of integration sites for the element in the staphylococcal chromosome. Based upon the unusually high rate of tryptophan auxotypy observed for TSST-1-producing strains, it has been suggested that this operon may be a preferred insertion site (CHU et al. 1985). Several classes of toxigenic clonal derivatives have been

```
1                                            11
MET ASN LYS LYS LEU LEU MET ASN PHE PHE ILE VAL SER PRO LEU


               21
LEU LEU ALA THR THR ALA THR ASP PHE THR PRO VAL PRO LEU SER

31                                           41
SER ASN GLN ILE ILE LYS THR ALA LYS ALA SER THR ASN ASP ASN

               51
ILE LYS ASP LEU LEU ASP TRP TYR SER SER GLY SER ASP THR PHE

61                                           71
THR ASN SER GLU VAL LEU ASP ASN SER LEU GLY SER MET ARG ILE

               81
LYS ASN THR ASP GLY SER ILE SER LEU ILE ILE PHE PRO SER PRO

91                                           101
TYR TYR SER PRO ALA PHE THR LYS GLY GLU LYS VAL ASP LEU ASN

               111
THR LYS ARG THR LYS LYS SER GLN HIS THR SER GLU GLY THR TYR

121                                          131
ILE HIS PHE GLN ILE SER GLY VAL THR ASN THR GLU LYS LEU PRO

               141
THR PRO ILE GLU LEU PRO LEU LYS VAL LYS VAL HIS GLY LYS ASP

151                                          161
SER PRO LEU LYS TYR GLY PRO LYS PHE ASP LYS LYS GLN LEU ALA

               171
ILE SER THR LEU ASP PHE GLU ILE ARG HIS GLN LEU THR GLN ILE

181                                          191
HIS GLY LEU TYR ARG SER SER ASP LYS THR GLY GLY TYR TRP LYS

               201
ILE THR MET ASN ASP GLY SER THR TYR GLN SER ASP LEU SER LYS

211                                          221
LYS PHE GLU TYR ASN THR GLU LYS PRO PRO ILE ASN ILE ASP GLU

               231
ILE LYS THR ILE GLU ALA GLU ILE ASN ***
```

Fig. 1. Amino acid sequence of TSST-1. Ser-41 is the first amino acid of the mature TSST-1 protein after cleavage of the signal peptide (residues 1–40)

identified based upon phenotypic and Southern hybridization analysis (KREISWIRTH et al. 1989; MUSSER et al. 1990). Restriction enzyme-digested DNA from a variety of clonal types produced several distinct hybridization patterns. Variability in profiles occurred even within the group of tryptophan auxotrophs.

tst expression appears to be regulated by one or more trans-acting regulatory elements which control expression of several S. aureus exoproteins. Insertion of transposon Tn551 into the S. aureus chromosome had a pleiotropic effect on expression of a variety of extracellular products, including a 30- to 40-fold decreased production of TSST-1 (RECSEI et al. 1985). Several other exoproteins including hemolysins (α, β, and δ) and staphylokinase also exhibited decreased production. In contrast, secreted protein A levels were elevated. Using northern blot analysis, the pleiotropic effect was shown to act at the level of transcription (RECSEI et al. 1986). This regulatory element, mapped between the purine B (purB) and isoleucine-valine (ilv) loci, was designated as accessory gene regulator or agr (RECSEI et al. 1985).

To confirm the trans-acting nature of agr, tst was transformed into the mutant strain on a high copy number plasmid (RECSEI et al. 1986). The mutant strain was unable to express either the cloned TSST-1 gene or the chromosome gene, indicating that the transposon had inactivated a trans-acting positive control element.

Subsequently, PENG et al. (1988) described the cloning and sequencing of agr. The gene was cloned initially in E. coli using an inserted transposon Tn551 as a cloning probe. Nucleotide sequencing revealed a 241-codon open reading frame containing the transposon insertion site. The cloned gene was recloned to an S. aureus vector, pSK265, and shown to be functional in S. aureus. Activity was evaluated by determination of α-hemolysin, β-hemolysin, and TSST-1 production in early stationary phase culture. The cloned gene exhibited considerable variation with respect to different exoproteins and different host strains compared to the chromosomal agr determinant (PENG et al. 1988). This complex pattern of expression probably will be understood completely only when the entire regulatory system is resolved.

Working independently, JANZON et al. (1986) subsequently described the same or similar regulatory element as agr by mutagenesis of a chromosome locus designated exp. The investigators found the regulatory effects of exp to be similar to that of agr. In addition, they reported positive exp regulation of serine and metalloproteases, nucleases, and acid phosphatase, and negative control of coagulase. The exp locus was identified using Tn551, cloned in E. coli, and shown to code for a 3.5 kb RNA species.

Recent studies have indicated that the mRNA from the δ toxin gene is important in agr control of toxin production.

TSST-1 has never been conclusively demonstrated to be produced by coagulase-negative S. aureus isolates (KREISWIRTH et al. 1987b). A large and diverse group of coagulase-negative staphylococci were assayed for the ability to produce TSST-1 by immunological reactivity and also to hybridize with a

TSST-1-specific gene probe. None of the coagulase-negative strains tested produced TSST-1, and no DNA homology was found with the gene probe.

The expression of *tst* is dependent on temperature, oxygen, and glucose level (SCHLIEVERT and BLOMSTER 1983) and can be significantly altered by submicrobicidal concentrations of clindamycin (SCHLIEVERT and KELLY 1984). Significantly more TSST-1 was made at 37 °C, rather than at 30 °C, although bacterial growth was similar at the two temperatures. Furthermore, toxin was made aerobically and not anaerobically in spite of only a twofold difference in bacterial growth. This has led to the theory that oxygen is an essential factor provided by the use of tampons explaining their association with TSS. *tst* expression was susceptible to catabolite repression by glucose. Glucose suppressed bacterial growth and, more extensively, toxin production at a level of 3% (w/v) glucose (SCHLIEVERT and BLOMSTER 1983). Clindamycin, an inhibitor of protein synthesis, completely inhibited production of TSST-1 at antibiotic concentrations that did not affect *S. aureus* growth (SCHLIEVERT and KELLY 1984).

3 Staphylococcal Enterotoxins B, C1, C2, and C3

The SEB gene, designated *entB*, was cloned in *E. coli* and sequenced by Khan and colleagues (RANELLI et al. 1985; JONES and KHAN 1986). The *entB* gene from chromosomal DNA of *S. aureus* strain S6 (DYER and IANDOLO 1981) was ligated to pBR322 and transformed into *E. coli* HB101 (RANELLI et al. 1985). Positive clones were selected by colony hybridization, but, surprisingly, the *E. coli* clones failed to produce SEB. When the *entB* gene was placed downstream from the strong L phage promotor, L_R, SEB production was detectable in *E. coli*, with mature protein almost exclusively present in the cytoplasmic fraction. The *entB* gene also was reintroduced into *S. aureus* RN4220 with pC193 as the vector, and the clones were shown to produce SEB.

Nucleotide sequencing determined the *entB* structural gene to be 798 nucleotides, which encode a 266 amino acid residue SEB precursor (JONES and KHAN 1986). A signal sequence of 27 amino acid residues is present at the N-terminal end, leaving the mature SEB with 239 amino acids (Fig. 2). This corresponds to a molecular weight of 28 336, which is in good agreement with published results obtained with purified protein (HUANG and BERGDOLL 1970).

The genes for SEC1, SEC2, and SEC3 also have been cloned from staphylococcal chromosomes and sequenced. *entC1* from *S. aureus* strain MN DON was cloned and sequenced by BOHACH and SCHLIEVERT (1987a, b). *entC2* and *entC3* genes were cloned and sequenced from staphylococcal strains FRI361 and FRI913, respectively (BOHACH and SCHLIEVERT 1989; HOVDE et al. 1990). Each of the three *entC* genes encodes a protein of 266 amino acids, with the first 27 amino acids comprising the signal peptide (Fig. 2). Thus, each mature

```
spea : MENNKKVLKKMVFFVLVTFLGLTISQEVFAQQDPDP........SQLHRSSLVKNLQYIY
spec : -KKINIIK..I--IIT-I...-ISTYFTYH-..S-Skkdisnvk-D-LYAYT......-T
sea  : -KKTAFT-..LL-IA-TL...T-SPL.-NGSEKSEEinekdlrkKSELQGTALG--KQ--
seb. : -YKRLFISHVILI-A-IL...VISTPN-L-ESQ---kpdelhk.-SKFTGLM.E-MKVL-
sec1 : -NKSRFISCVILI-A-IL...VLFTPN-L-ESQ---tpdelhk.ASKFTGLM.E-MKVL-
sec2 : -NKSRFISCVILI-A-IL...VLFTPN-L-ESQ---tpdelhk.-SEFTGTM.G-MK-L-
sec3 : -YKRLFISRVILI-A-IL...VISTPN-L-ESQ---mpddlhk.-SEFTGTM.G-MK-L-
sed  : -KKFNILI..ALL-FTSL...VISPLN-K-NENI-SvkekelhkKSELS-TALN-MKHS-
see  : -KKTAFI-..LL-IA-TL...T-SPL.-NGSEKSEEinekdlrkKSELQRNALS--RQ--

spea : FLYEGDPVTHENVKSVDQLLSHDLIYNVSG...PNYDKLKTELKNQEMATLFKDKNV.DI
spec : PYDYK-CR..V-FSTTHT-NIDTQK-RGKDyyiSSEM.......SY-ASQK--RDDHv-V
sea  : YYN-KAKT..--KE-H--F-Q-TILFKGFFtdhSW-ND-LVDFDSKDIVDKY-G-Kv.-L
seb  : DDNHVSAI..NVKSID.-F-YF----SIKDtklG---NVRV-F--KDL-DKY-.DKYv-V
sec1 : DDHYVSAT..KVKSVD.KF-A------I-DkklK----V----L-EGL-KKY-.DE-v-V
sec2 : DDHYVSAT..KVMSVD.KF-A------I-DkklK----V----L-EDL-KKY-.DE-v-V
sec3 : DDHYVSAT..KVKSVD.KF-A------I-DkklK----V----L-EDL-KKY-.DE-v-V
sed  : ADKNPIIG..--KSTG--F-ENT-L-KKFFtdlI-FED-LINFNSK---QH--S--v.-V
see  : YYN-KAIT..--KE-D--F-ENT-LFKGFFtgh-W-ND-LVD-GSKDATNKY-G-Kv.-L

spea : YGVEYYHLCYLCENAE.........RSACIYGGVTNHEGNHLEILKKIVVKV..SIDGIQ
spec : F-LF-ILNSHtgeyi.............---I-PAQN-KVNH..-L..LGnlF-S-ES
sea  : --AY-GYQ-Aggtpn..........KT--M-----L-DN-R-TEE--V..PInlWL--K-
seb  : F-AN---YQ--FSKKTNdinshqtdk-KT-M-----E-N--Q-DKYRS-T-rv..FE--KN
sec1 : --SN--VN--FSSKDNvgkvtgg...KT-M---I-K-----FDNGNLQN-LIrvYENKRN
sec2 : --SN--VN--FSSKDNvgkvtgg...KT-M---I-K-----FDNGNLQN-LIrvYENKRN
sec3 : --SN--VN--FSSKDNvgkvtgg...KT-M---I-K-----FDNGNLQN-L-rvYENKRN
sed  : -PIR-SIN--ggeid..........-T--T-----F----K-KER---..PInlW-N-V-
see  : --AY-GYQ-Aggtpn..........KT--M-----L-DN-R-TEE--V..PInlW---K-

spea : S..LSFDIETNKKMVTAQELDYKVRKYLTDNKQLYTNGPSKYET...GYIKFIPKNKESF
spec : Qqn-NNK-ILE-DI--F--I-F-I----M--YKI-D.AT-P-VS...-R-EIGT-DGKHE
sea  : NtvPLETVK----N--V----LQA-R--QEKYN--N.SDVFDGKvqr-L-V-HTSTEP-V
seb  : L..----VQ----K--------LT-H--VK--K--EFNN-P---...------ENE.N--
sec1 : T..I--EVQ-D--S-------I-A-NF-INK-N--EFNS-P---...------EN-GNT-
sec2 : T..I--EVQ-D--S-------I-A-NF-INK-N--EFNS-P---...------EN-GNT-
sec3 : T..I--EVQ-D--S-------I-A-NF-INK-N--EFNS-P---...------EN-GNT-
sed  : KevSLDKVQ-D--N--V----AQA-R--QKDLK--N.NDTLGGKiqr-K-E-DSSDGSKV
see  : TtvPIDKVK-S--E--V----LQA-H--HGKFG--N.SD-FGGKvqr-L-V-HSSEGSTV

spea : WFDFFPE.P.....EFTQSKYLMIYKDNETLDS.NTSQIEVYLTTK@
spec : QI-L-DSpn.....-G-R-DIFAK----RIINMk-F-HFDI--.E--
sea  : NY-L-GA.QqqysnTLLRI.....-R--K-IN-e-M.H-DI--Y-S-
seb  : -Y-MM-A.-gdkfdQ...-----M-N--KMV--kDVK.-------K
sec1 : -Y-MM-A.-gdkfdQ...-----M-N--K-V--kSVK.---H----N
sec2 : -Y-MM-A.-gdkfdQ...-----M-N--K-V--kSVK.---H----N
sec3 : -Y-MM-A.-gdkfdQ...-----M-N--K-V--kSVK.---H----N
sed  : SY-L-DV.KgdfpeKQLRI.....-S--K--STeHL.H-DI--YE--
see  : SY-L-DA.QgqypdTLLRI.....-R--K-IN-e-L.H-DL--Y-T-
```

Fig. 2. Single letter amino acid sequence of SPE A and C and SEs A–E aligned using the Molecular Biology Information Resource (MBIR) programs from the Department of Cell Biology, Baylor College of Medicine, Houston, TX. Sequences include the signal peptide for each toxin and are aligned in reference to SPE A. *Dashes* indicate sequence identity with SPE A; *dots* indicate gaps in the sequence to obtain optimal alignment; *upper case letters* refer to aligned nonidentical amino acids with SPE A; *lower case letters* refer to unaligned amino acids

SEC protein is comprised of 239 amino acids with a molecular weight of 27 563. The mature SEC1 and SEC2 proteins differ at seven amino acid positions, all in the N-terminal half, as determined by nucleotide and amino acid sequencing. Four of the differences result in charge differences and explain the isoelectric point difference between SEC1 (pl 8.5) and SEC2 (pl 7.0). The SEC3 signal peptide is considerably different from that of SEC1 and SEC2 but is nearly identical to that of SEB. The mature SEC3 protein differs from the other SECs at a number of amino acid positions, but again the differences are primarily in the N-terminal end. SEC3 differs from SEC1 by nine amino acid residues and from SEC2 by four residues. The 167 C-terminal residues of the three SECs are identical, except for one conservative amino acid substitution in SEC3.

Unlike SEB expression in *E. coli*, SECs are expressed from their promoters (RANELLI et al. 1985; BOHACH and SCHLIEVERT 1987a, 1989; HOVDE et al. 1990). Since SEC1 and SEB putative promoter regions differ by only one nucleotide (JONES and KHAN 1986; BOHACH and SCHLIEVERT 1987b), it is likely that the failure of expression of SEB initially in *E. coli* by RANELLI et al. (1985) was the result of catabolite repression rather than failure to promote. Indeed, our studies indicate cloned SEB is expressible in the absence of glucose but is easily repressed by even small amounts of glucose.

The shared biological and immunological properties of most members of the pyrogenic toxin family appear to be a direct consequence of sequence similarity at the molecular level (Fig. 2). SCHMIDT and SPERO (1983) first demonstrated that SEB and SEC1 possessed significant amino acid similarity, despite their immunological distinction. Subsequently, sequence analysis of the SPE A, SEB, and SEC1 structural genes and computer alignment of their deduced primary sequences showed that all three toxins were related (JOHNSON et al. 1986a; JONES and KHAN 1986; WEEKS and FERRETTI 1986; BOHACH and SCHLIEVERT 1987b). The nucleotide sequence of *entC1* has 74% and 59% homology with the other two toxin genes, *entB* and *speA*, respectively (BOHACH and SCHLIEVERT 1987b). Amino acid homology, analyzed by computer alignment of the three proteins, was highly significant. Their C-terminal ends and sequences flanking the enterotoxin cysteine loop are most conserved among all three proteins (BOHACH and SCHLIEVERT 1987b). The SEB and SEC1 sequences are also highly similar in their N-terminals, whereas the SPE A sequence is quite different in this part of the molecule.

Likewise, the degree of immunological relatedness among the three types of SECs appears to be proportional to their molecular relatedness. HOVDE et al. (1990) also have provided evidence that the N-terminals of SECs determine subtype-specific antigenic epitopes, while the more conserved C-terminal regions determine biological properties and cross-reactive antigenic epitopes shared with other pyrogenic toxins.

Although genetic systems for the staphylococcal enterotoxins are diverse, some similarities have been demonstrated among *entB* and *entC*s. One study, primarily on SEB producers, suggested that *entB* is transferred by a hitchhiking transposon (NOVICK et al. 1980). In these systems, the mobile gene on a site-specific element has a high transposition frequency. The transposition onto a carrier plasmid is required for mobilization. Evidence suggested that SEC1 element is under similar regulation.

Several conflicting reports concerning the genomic location and mechanism of *entB* mobility suggested that the genetic system involved is complex. Initial studies provided evidence that *entB* in hospital isolates was plasmid borne and yet is linked to a chromosomal determinant for methicillin resistance (*mec*) (DORNBUSCH 1971; SHALITA et al. 1977). A later investigation demonstrated a chromosomal location for *entB* in food poisoning isolates (SHAFER and IANDOLO 1978a). SHAFER and IANDOLO (1979) later reported that *entB* may be harbored on either the chromosome or a plasmid. Although transiently associated with *mec*, the two genes were not physically linked. Evidence for the role of a small staphylococcal plasmid (pSN2) in regulation of *entB* expression (DYER and IANDOLO 1981) was disputed by the results of KHAN and NOVICK (1982).

Southern hybridization using toxin gene probes revealed a high degree of restriction length polymorphism for *entB* and *entC1*. In one report the *entB* locus was suggested to be invariable (RANELLI et al. 1985). However, subsequent study of a large number of toxigenic strains from a variety of sources revealed numerous clonal variations based on toxin profiles and probing results (BOHACH et al. 1989). Human strains that were TSST-1-negative had extensive restriction length polymorphism for *entC1*. In contrast, strains that coproduced TSST-1 and SEC1 displayed little variability, although human and animal strains had clearly distinct hybridization patterns. Strains which coproduce SEB and SEC1 are rare. However, in at least one strain, both genes are harbored on the same plasmid (ALTBOUM et al. 1985). This plasmid, which also encodes methicillin resistance, occasionally integrates into the chromosome.

The combined current evidence suggests that TSST-1, SEB, and SECs are contained on mobile genetic elements, similar to hitchhiking transposons described previously (NOVICK et al. 1980). Presumably, these elements have a limited number of preferred integration sites, which could explain several observations including restriction length variability, the influence of *tst* on *entC1* probing profiles, and the mutually exclusive occurrence or rarity of some toxin combinations (TSST-1 and SEB; SEC1 and SEB) (BOHACH et al. 1990).

Lastly, similar to TSST-1, recent studies have revealed production of SPE A, SEB and SECs to be at least partially under *agr* control.

4 Staphylococcal Enterotoxins A, D, and E

Staphylococcal enterotoxin A has been cloned and sequenced by Betley and colleagues (BETLEY et al. 1984; BETLEY and MEKALANOS 1988). The *entA* gene was isolated from the chromosome of *S. aureus* strain FRI337, ligated to pBR322, and transformed into *E. coli* AB259 (MURRAY et al. 1973; BETLEY et al. 1984).

Mature SEA was expressed and determined to be secreted into the periplasmic space of *E. coli*.

Nucleotide sequencing showed *entA* to be 771 bp thus encoding an SEA precursor protein (Fig. 2) of 257 amino acids (BETLEY and MEKALANOS 1988). The first 24 residues of the N-terminal represents the hydrophobic leader sequence that is processed, leaving the mature SEA protein with 233 amino acids (molecular weight 27 100). Sequence comparison of SEA to the SEs revealed about 23% amino acid homology with SEB and SEC1 (BETLEY and MEKALANOS, 1988).

SHAFER and IANDOLO (1978b) reported that the *entA* gene is located on the chromosome from examining two well-known SEA-positive *S. aureus* strains, FRI100 and S6. Strain FRI100 lacks any extrachromosomal DNA and strain S6 still made SEA after being cured of its single plasmid. Furthermore, in 24 of 29 SEA-positive strains tested, the *entA* gene was mapped between the *pur* and *ilv* markers in the chromosome (MALLONEE et al. 1982; PATTEE and GLATZ 1980). In the remaining five strains, *entA* gene was not found in any of the previously mapped chromosomal linkage groups (MALLONEE et al. 1982).

Using DNA hybridization analysis with a cloned *entA* gene, BETLEY et al. (1984) showed that the toxin gene-containing element was detected in at least two chromosomal locations. They believe that this heterologous insertion site may be a "hotspot for structural rearrangement." Also, the *entA* structural gene, and not the regulatory element, is linked to the *pur-ilv* region in some SEA-positive strains. The *entA* gene appears to be part of an 8-12 kb genetic element (BETLEY et al. 1984).

An early study of SEA-positive strain PS42-D described the presence of prophage (CASMAN 1965). BETLEY and MEKALANOS (1985) later confirmed that *entA* gene is phage-associated in all positive strains examined. Viable *entA*-converting phages were isolated from two different wild-type SEA-positive strains. One of the phages contains a 49 kb DNA with the *entA* gene being near the phage attachment site. DNA hybridization showed that *entA* gene is associated with phage-related DNA in all strains examined. Some *entA* genes were associated with either defective phage or phage with altered host range, and plaque-forming units were not isolated from at least one toxin-positive strain.

The SED structural gene has been cloned and sequenced by BAYLES and IANDOLO (1989). *entD* was shown to reside on a 27.6 kb penicillinase plasmid designated pIB485 from SED-positive *S. aureus* strain KSI1410. *entD* gene was isolated and ligated to pBR322 and transformed into *E. coli* LE392. The transformants expressed SED as determined by western blot analysis.

Nucleotide sequencing of *entD* revealed an open reading frame of 774 bp, encoding a 258 amino acid precursor protein (BAYLES and IANDOLO 1989). The first 30 amino acids represented the signal peptide, leaving the mature protein (Fig. 2) with 228 residues and a molecular weight of 26 360. This is close to the previous SDS-PAGE determined molecular weight of 27 300 (CHANG and BERGDOLL 1979). Comparison of amino acid sequences showed that SED shared between 53.1% and 55.0% sequence identity with SEA and SEE and only near 40% identity with SEB, SEC1, and SPE A (BAYLES and IANDOLO 1989). Two regions of SED (from residue 101 to 114 and from 142 to 158) are highly homologous to other SEs and appear to be conserved among all SEs.

As mentioned, *entD* gene was localized on a penicillinase plasmid (BAYLES and IANDOLO 1989). This plasmid was found in all SED-producing strains examined. The presence of toxin gene-containing plasmids or other unique elements appears to be fairly common in *S. aureus*. For example, both structural genes for SEB and SEC1 (ALTBOUM et al. 1985) and the gene encoding exfoliative toxin B (WARREN et al. 1975) can be plasmid-associated in *S. aureus*.

BAYLES and IANDOLO (1989) identified two regions upstream from *entD* that may play important roles. First, S1 nuclease protection analysis indicated that transcription is initiated 266 nucleotides upstream from the *entD* translation start codon. Second, an inverted repeat sequence was discovered which resembles similar regions identified upstream of other staphylococcal extracellular protein genes (JONES and KHAN 1986; LEE and IANDOLO 1986; LEE et al. 1987; O'TOOLE and FOSTER 1987; SHORTLE 1983). These also have similar arm lengths of 12–14 bp. The role of the inverted repeat sequence upstream from *entD* is uncertain. One possibility is transcriptional regulation since a similar inverted repeat sequence is located upstream from the transcription start site of *entB* (GASKILL and KHAN 1988). This regulation is possibly due to *agr* which already has been shown to regulate the expression of *tst*, *entB*, and *entC*s. Interestingly, SEA does not appear to be under *agr* control.

The *entE* gene was cloned and sequenced by COUCH et al. (1988). The *entE* gene was isolated from *S. aureus* strain FRI198, ligated to pBR322, and introduced into *E. coli* 259 (MURRAY et al. 1973). SEE produced by the *E. coli* clone was serologically identical to SEE produced by *S. aureus*. Sequencing analysis revealed the *entE* structural gene to contain 771 bp, encoding a precursor protein (Fig. 2) of 257 amino acid residues. N-terminal amino acid sequencing revealed that a signal peptide of 27 amino acids is cleaved, resulting in a 230 residue mature SEE with a molecular weight of 26 425. The comparison of *entE* nucleotide sequence with other related toxin genes showed that the former exhibited 84% homology with *entA* and 52%, 50%, and 51% homology with *entB*, *entC1*, and *speA*, respectively. Thus far, *entE* has not been shown to be phage-associated (COUCH et al. 1988).

5 Streptococcal Pyrogenic Exotoxins Types A and C

Group A streptococcal pyrogenic exotoxin type A was cloned from the bacteriophage T12 genome by JOHNSON and SCHLIEVERT (1984) and was sequenced by WEEKS and FERRETTI (1986) and JOHNSON et al. (1986a). In cloning *speA*, the gene was localized onto a 1.75 kb *SalI-HindIII* restriction endonuclease fragment, ligated to pBR322 vector, and transformed into *E. coli*. The cloned toxin expressed in *E. coli* migrated as two bands, comparable to that derived from streptococci, and was biochemically, biologically, and immunologically related to native SPE A (JOHNSON and SCHLIEVERT 1984). WEEKS and FERRETTI (1984) confirmed these findings in similar studies.

The *speA* gene has been expressed in a variety of backgrounds. Following initial cloning in *E. coli*, the gene was cloned on a high copy number plasmid in *B. subtilis* in an attempt to facilitate large-scale toxin production (KREISWIRTH et al. 1987a). *Bacillus* produced 32-fold more SPE A than the native streptococcus; however, difficulties were encountered in resolubilization of the purified and cloned protein. This problem was avoided when *speA* was cloned into *S. aureus* RN4220 using pBR328-pE194 chimeric cloning vector. The toxin gene has also been cloned into *Streptococcus sanguis* (WEEKS and FERRETTI 1984).

Nucleotide sequencing analysis of *speA* gene by WEEKS and FERRETTI (1986) and by JOHNSON et al. (1986a) determined SPE A to consist of 251 amino acids (Fig. 2) of which the first 30 comprise a signal peptide. At the 3' end of the *speA* gene, there are two inverted repeat sequences that are required for toxin expression; these sequences were proposed to provide a stem and loop structure necessary to stabilize the message.

Sequence comparisons of SPE A with other related pyrogenic toxins have revealed significant sequence homology with staphylococcal toxins SEB and SECs (JOHNSON et al. 1986a; BOHACH and SCHLIEVERT 1987b, 1989; HOVDE et al. 1990). Thus, it has been proposed that these toxins, which share numerous biological activities, may have similar active site structures.

It has long been suspected that SPE A may be phage-encoded and that bacteriophage and lysogeny were important in regulation and transfer of SPE A. In 1927, FROBISHER and BROWN reported that a filterable agent from toxigenic group A streptococci could confer toxigenicity to nontoxigenic strains. This was confirmed later by BINGEL (1949) and by ZABRISKIE (1964), who demonstrated that a lysogenic bacteriophage was responsible for this earlier observation. Zabriske showed that infection of *S. pyogenes* strain T25$_3$ with phage from strain T12gl resulted in a lysogenic strain T25$_3$(T12gl) with ability to produce SPE. Phage curing techniques promoted loss of toxigenicity. Others subsequently have confirmed these findings (NIDA et al. 1979; JOHNSON et al. 1980; McKANE and FERRETTI 1981; NIDA and FERRETTI 1982).

As mentioned above, JOHNSON and SCHLIEVERT (1983) later analyzed purified DNA from the lysogenic phage (T12) and showed that the genome was 36 kb in length, circularly permuted, and terminally redundant. They eventually confirmed that the SPE A structural gene was carried by phage T12 (JOHNSON and SCHLIEVERT 1984). JOHNSON et al. (1986b) have shown that the phage attachment site for incorporation into the bacterial genome mapped adjacent to *speA*, thus suggesting that phage T12 may have acquired the toxin gene from the bacterial genome by abnormal excision. DNA sequences similar to the phage DNA were common in nontoxigenic strains. All SPE A-positive strains tested carried both *speA* and phage T12 sequences adjacent to each other, suggesting that *speA* is phage-encoded. Although *speA* is now a permanent component of the T12 phage genome, converting phage were not induced from a high percentage of toxigenic strains (JOHNSON et al. 1986b). These strains harbored heterogeneous remnants of the phage genome adjacent to *speA*, and presumably the phages are defective and have lost their excision capability.

In recent studies, *speA* and SPE A have been associated with development of toxic shock-like syndrome (TSLS). In 1987 CONE et al. identified a SPE A-producing streptococcal strain from one of two patients with TSLS. Subsequently, nine of ten isolates were reported to make SPE A in association with cases of TSLS from the western United States (STEVENS et al. 1989). Most recently, HAUSER et al. (1990) examined 34 streptococcal strains isolated from patients with clinically well-documented TSLS (M type) and a pyrogenic toxin profile. Of the isolates, 74% were of either M type 1 or 3, with the remainder being scattered among several other M types. It was determined that 53% produced SPE A as detected by Ouchterlony immunodiffusion and that 85% contained the *speA* gene as determined by Southern hybridization. These figures are in contrast with the published value of 15% for the incidence of *speA* in group A streptococcal isolates in general (YU and FERRETTI 1989). It was concluded that SPE A may have an important causal role in TSLS.

HAUSER et al. (1990) also showed that *speA* restriction fragment length polymorphism (RFLP) is constant within an M type but is different between M types. Thus, M type 1 isolates of group A streptococci associated with TSLS contained *speA* on a 14 kb *Pst*I fragment, whereas M type 3 isolates contained *speA* on a 23 kb *Pst*I fragment. It was proposed that *spe* RFLP may be useful as an adjunct to M typing in categorizing and determining relatedness of streptococcal isolates.

The structural gene of SPE C was cloned initially from the chromosome of *S. pyogenes* strain T18P into *E. coli* using pBR328 as the vector plasmid (GOSHORN et al. 1988). Partially purified *E. coli*-derived SPE C and purified streptococcal-derived toxin were shown to have the same molecular weight and biological activities. As with SPE A structural gene, when SPE C gene was recloned into *S. aureus* RN4220, the transformants were able to express mature SPE C.

Nucleotide sequencing of *speC* produced an open reading frame of 705 bp coding for 235 amino acid residues (GOSHORN and SCHLIEVERT 1988). After cleavage of the 27 amino acid signal peptide, mature SPE C protein (Fig. 2) was determined to be 208 amino acid residues, with a calculated molecular weight of 24 354. Comparison of the *speC* nucleotide sequence to other related toxins' sequences revealed the greatest amount of homology with the 3' end of *speA*.

JOHNSON et al. (1980) and COLON-WHITT et al. (1979) first demonstrated that SPE C production in *S. pyogenes* was transferred by lysogenic conversion. These reports were confirmed by other independent investigators (NIDA and FERRETTI 1982). Hybridization experiments confirmed that the *speC* structural gene was located on the CS112 bacteriophage genome of SPE C-producing streptococci (GOSHORN et al. 1988). Genetic factors involved in SPE C production appeared similar to those described previously for SPE A and staphylococcal SEA (BETLEY and MEKALANOS 1985). First, it was not possible to induce toxin-converting phage from most group A streptococcal strains that produce SPE C. In addition, as described for *speA*, *speC* mapped closely to the phage attachment site (GOSHORN and SCHLIEVERT 1989) and thus was probably acquired from the bacterial genome by abnormal excision.

Recently, HAUSER et al. (1990) demonstrated that *speC* was present in 21% of TSLS-associated streptococci.

6 Streptococcal Pyrogenic Exotoxin Type B

The structural gene encoding SPE B, designated *speB*, was cloned from the chromosome of group A streptococcal strain 86-858 (which contains *speB* but not *speA* or *speC*) into *E. coli* (BOHACH et al. 1988). Toxin prepared from the *E. coli* clone was biochemically and biologically similar to streptococcal-derived toxin. After further subcloning and gene localization studies, *speB* was sequenced and the resultant amino acid sequence was compared to two different N-terminal partial amino acid sequences (HAUSER and SCHLIEVERT 1990).

speB consisted of an 1194 base pair open reading frame encoding a 398 amino acid protein that contained a 27 residue signal peptide not present on the mature toxin (Fig. 3). The mature protein (371 residues, molecular weight 40 314) was subsequently proteolyzed to yield a 253 residue cleavage product (molecular weight 27 580). N-terminal amino acid sequencing of the native and proteolyzed SPE B confirmed the location of the cleavage site and that processing of native toxin had occurred. Interestingly, SPE B is the only member of the pyrogenic toxin that undergoes this processing.

Comparison of the inferred amino acid sequence of SPE B with other pyrogenic toxins revealed minimal sequence similarity, with only TSST-1 having possible relatedness to SPE B as determined by Monte Carlo analysis. SPE B, however, has highly significant sequence similarity with streptococcal pro-teinase precursor (SPP), a cysteine protease elaborated by group A streptococci as a zymogen that is activated upon reduction. Surprisingly, SPE B, as isolated from strain 86–858, was shown to be proteolytically inactive by use of a highly sensitive fluorescence assay. An explanation for the lack of protease activity of SPE B may be the rearrangement of amino acids of the active center compared to SPP. SPE B and SPP have been shown to share biological activities which typify pyrogenic exotoxins.

In subsequent studies, it was shown by Southern hybridization analysis with use of an internal *speB* probe that all group A streptococci contain one *speB* gene (HAUSER and SCHLIEVERT 1990; HAUSER et al. 1990). This finding is significant for three reasons: (1) Only approximately 50% of group A streptococci elaborate SPE B even though all contain the *speB* gene. Thus, there must be some regulatory element influencing expression of *speB* or posttranslationally

```
1                                                11
MET ASN LYS LYS LYS LEU GLY ILE ARG LEU LEU SER LEU LEU ALA
                                                 (1)
              21                                  ↓
LEU GLY GLY PHE VAL LEU ALA ASN PRO VAL PHE ALA ASP GLN ASN

31                                      41
PHE ALA ARG ASN GLU LYS GLU ALA LYS ASP SER ALA ILE THR PHE

              51
ILE GLN LYS SER ALA ALA ILE LYS ALA GLY ALA ARG SER ALA GLU

61                                      71
ASP ILE LYS LEU ASP LYS VAL ASN LEU GLY GLY GLU LEU SER GLY

              81
SER ASN MET TYR VAL TYR ASN ILE SER THR GLY GLY PHE VAL ILE

91                                      101
VAL SER GLY ASP LYS ARG SER PRO GLU ILE LEU GLY TYR SER THR

              111
SER GLY SER PHE ASP ALA ASN GLY LYS GLU ASN ILE ALA SER PHE

121                                     131
MET GLU SER TYR VAL GLU GLN ILE LYS GLU ASN LYS LYS LEU ASP
                                    (2)
              141                    ↓
THR THR TYR ALA GLY THR ALA GLU ILE LYS GLN PRO VAL VAL LYS

151                                     161
SER LEU LEU ASP SER LYS GLY ILE HIS TYR ASN GLN GLY ASN PRO

              171
TYR ASN LEU LEU THR PRO VAL ILE GLU LYS VAL LYS PRO GLY GLU

181                                     191
GLN SER PHE VAL GLY GLN HIS ALA ALA THR GLY CYS VAL ALA THR

              201
ALA THR ALA GLN ILE MET LYS TYR HIS ASN TYR PRO ASN LYS GLY

211                                     221
LEU LYS ASP TYR THR TYR THR LEU SER SER ASN ASN PRO TYR PHE

              231
ASN HIS PRO LYS ASN LEU PHE ALA ALA ILE SER THR ARG GLN TYR

241                                     251
ASN TRP ASN ASN ILE LEU PRO THR TYR SER GLY ARG GLU SER ASN

              261
VAL GLN LYS MET ALA ILE SER GLU LEU MET ALA ASP VAL GLY ILE

271                                     281
SER VAL ASP MET ASP TYR GLY PRO SER SER GLY SER ALA GLY SER

              291
SER ARG VAL GLN ARG ALA LEU LYS GLU ASN PHE GLY TYR ASN GLN

301                                     311
SER VAL HIS GLN ILE ASN ARG SER ASP PHE SER LYS GLN ASP TRP
```

Fig. 3 (Continued)

```
          321
GLU ALA GLN ILE ASP LYS GLU LEU SER GLN ASN GLN PRO VAL TYR

331                           341
TYR GLN GLY VAL GLY LYS VAL GLY GLY HIS ALA PHE VAL ILE ASP

          351
GLY ALA ASP GLY ARG ASN PHE TYR HIS VAL ASN TRP GLY TRP GLY

361                           371
GLY VAL SER ASP GLY PHE PHE ARG LEU ASP ALA LEU ASN PRO SER

          381
ALA LEU GLY THR GLY GLY GLY ALA GLY GLY PHE ASN GLY TYR GLN

391
SER ALA VAL VAL GLY ILE LYS PRO ***
```

Fig. 3. Amino acid sequence of SPE B. *Arrows* indicate the cleavage sites for removal of the signal peptide (*1*) and for generation of the final stable SPE B product (*2*)

modifying the toxin protein (2) SPE B and SPP share greater than 90% amino acid sequence similarity and thus most certainly should contain highly significant nucleotide sequence relatedness. The observation that the *speB* probe hybridizes to only one gene suggests more strongly that SPE B and SPP are encoded by the same gene. (3) Previously, it was suggested that SPE B production was transferrable from one streptococcal strain to another by bacteriophage. Since *speB* is not a viable trait in streptococci, it is highly unlikely that the *speB* gene is carried by bacteriophage (in contrast to *speA* and *speC*). Therefore, the bacteriophage must have been positively influencing *speB* expression.

Recent studies have shown that all TSLS isolates of group A streptococci, like group A strains from other sources, contain the *speB* gene, yet only 59% make the toxin, again similar to non-TSLS strains (HAUSER et al. 1990). Thus, SPE B is not specifically associated with TSLS. *speB* present in TSLS isolates was contained on the same *Pst*I restriction enzyme digesting fragment within an M type of group A streptococcus, but different M types contained *speB* on different size DNA fragments.

References

Altboum Z, Hertman I, Sarid S (1985) Penicillinase plasmid-linked genetic determinants for enterotoxins B and C1 production in *Staphylococcus aureus*. Infect Immun 47: 514–521

Bayles KW, Iandolo JJ (1989) Genetic and molecular analysis of the gene encoding staphylococcal enterotoxin D. J Bacteriol 171: 4799–4806

Betley MJ, Mekalanos JJ (1985) Staphylococcal enterotoxin A is encoded by phage. Science 229: 185–187

Betley MJ, Mekalanos JJ (1988) Nucleotide sequence of the type A staphylococcal enterotoxin gene. J Bacteriol 170: 34–41

Betley MJ, Lofdahl S, Kreiswirth BN, Bergdoll MS, Novick RP (1984) Staphylococcal enterotoxin A gene is associated with a variable genetic determinant. Proc Natl Acad Sci USA 81: 5179–5183

Bingel KF (1949) Neue Untersuchungen zur Scharlachätiologie. Dsch Med Woch 127: 703–706

Blomster-Hautamaa DA, Kreiswirth BN, Novick RP, Schlievert PM (1986a) Resolution of highly purified toxic-shock syndrome toxin-1 into two distinct proteins by isoelectric focusing. Biochemistry 25: 54–59

Blomster-Hautamaa DA, Kreiswirth BN, Kornblum JS, Novick RP, Schlievert PM (1986b) The nucleotide and partial amino acid sequence of toxic shock syndrome toxin-1. J Biol Chem 261: 15783–15786

Bohach GA, Schlievert PM (1987a) Expression of staphylococcal enterotoxin C1 in *Escherichia coli*. Infect Immun 55: 428–432

Bohach GA, Schlievert PM (1987b) Nucleotide sequence of the staphylococcal enterotoxin C1 gene and relatedness to other pyrogenic toxins. Mol Gen Genet 209: 15–20

Bohach GA, Schlievert PM (1989) Conservation of the biologically-active portions of staphylococcal enterotoxins C1 and C2. Infect Immun 57: 2249–2252

Bohach GA, Hauser AR, Schlievert PM (1988) Cloning of the gene, *speB*, for streptococcal pyrogenic exotoxin type B in *Escherichia coli*. Infect Immun 56: 1665–1667

Bohach GA, Kreiswirth BN, Novick RP, Schlievert PM (1989) Analysis of toxic shock syndrome isolates producing staphylococcal enterotoxins B and C1 using southern hybridization and immunological assays. Rev Infect Dis 11: S75–S82

Bohach GA, Fast DJ, Nelson RD, Schlievert PM (1990) Staphylococcal and streptococcal pyrogenic toxins involved in toxic shock syndrome and related illnesses. Crit Rev Microbiol 17: 251–272

Casman EP (1965) Staphylococcal enterotoxin. Ann NY Acad Sci 128: 124–131

Chang PC, Bergdoll MS (1979) Purification and some physiochemical properties of staphylococcal enterotoxin D. Biochemistry 10: 1937–1942

Chu MC, Melish ME, James JM (1985) Tryptophan auxotypy associated with *Staphylococcus aureus* that produce toxic-shock syndrome toxin. J Infect Dis 151: 1157–1161

Colon-Whitt A, Whitt RS, Cole RM (1979) Production of an erythrogenic toxin (streptococcal pyrogenic exotoxin) by a nonlysogenized group A streptococcus. In: Parker MT (ed) Pathogenic streptococci. Reedbooks, Chertsey

Cone LA, Woodard DR, Schlievert PM, Tomory GS (1987) Clinical and bacteriologic observations of a toxic shock-like syndrome due to *Streptococcus pyogenes*. N Engl J Med 317: 146–149

Couch JL, Soltis MT, Betley MJ (1988) Cloning and nucleotide sequence of the type E staphylococcal enterotoxin gene. J Bacteriol 170: 2954–2960

Dornbusch K (1971) Genetic aspects of methicillin resistance and toxin production in a strain of *Staphylococcus aureus*. Ann NY Acad Sci 182: 91–97

Dyer DW, Iandolo JJ (1981) Plasmid-chromosomal transition of genes important in staphylococcal enterotoxin B expression. Infect Immun 33: 450–458

Frobisher M, Brown JH (1927) Transmissible toxigenicity of streptococci. Bull Johns Hopkins Hosp 41: 167–173

Gaskill ME, Khan SA (1988) Regulation of the enterotoxin B gene in *Staphylococcus aureus*. J Biol Chem 263: 6276–6280

Goshorn SC, Schlievert PM (1988) Nucleotide sequence of streptococcal pyrogenic exotoxin type C. Infect Immun 56: 2518–2520

Goshorn SC, Schlievert PM (1989) Bacteriophage association of streptococcal pyrogenic exotoxin type C. J Bacteriol 171: 3068–3073

Goshorn SC, Bohach GA, Schlievert PM (1988) Cloning and characterization of the gene, *speC*, for pyrogenic exotoxin type C from *Streptococcus pyogenes*. Mol Gen Genet 212: 66–70

Hauser AR, Schlievert PM (1990) Nucleotide sequence of the streptococcal pyrogenic exotoxin type B gene and relationship between the toxin and the streptococcal proteinase precursor. J Bacteriol 172: 4536–4542

Hauser AR, Stevens DL, Kaplan EL, Schlievert PM (1990) Molecular analysis of pyrogenic exotoxins from *Streptococcus pyogenes* isolates associated with toxic shock-like syndrome. J Clin Microbiol, in press

Horinouchi S, Weisblum (1982) Nucleotide sequence and functional map of pE194, a plasmid that specifies inducible resistance to macrolide, lincosamide, and streptogramin type B antibiotics. J Bacteriol 150: 804–814

Hovde CJ, Hackett SP, Bohach GA (1990) Nucleotide sequence of the staphylococcal enterotoxin C3 gene: sequence comparison of all three type C staphylococcal enterotoxins. Mol Gen Genet 220: 329–333

Huang IY, Bergdoll MS (1970) The primary structure of staphylococcal enterotoxin B. J Biol Chem 245: 3518–3525

Igarashi H, Fujikawa H, Usami H, Kawabata S, Morita T (1984) Purification and characterization of *Staphylococcus aureus* FRI1169 and 587 toxic shock syndrome exotoxins. Infect Immun 44: 175–181

Janzon L, Lofdahl S, Arvidson S (1986) Evidence for a coordinate transcriptional control of a alpha-toxin and protein A in *Staphylococcus aureus*. FEMS Microbiol Lett 33: 193–198

Johnson LP, Schlievert PM (1983) A physical map of the group A streptococcal pyrogenic exotoxin bacteriophage T12gI genome. Mol Gen Genet 189: 251–255

Johnson LP, Schlievert PM (1984) Group A streptococcal phage T12 carries the structural gene for pyrogenic exotoxin type A. Mol Gen Genet 194: 52–56

Johnson LP, Schlievert PM, Watson DW (1980) Transfer of group A streptococcal pyrogenic exotoxin production to nontoxigenic strains by lysogenic conversion. Infect Immun 28: 254–257

Johnson LP, L'Italien JJ, Schlievert PM (1986a) Streptococcal pyrogenic exotoxin type A (scarlet fever toxin) is related to *Staphylococcus aureus* enterotoxin B. Mol Gen Genet 203: 354–356

Johnson LP, Tomai MA, Schlievert PM (1986b) Bacteriophage involvement in group A streptococcal pyrogenic exotoxin A production. J Bacteriol 166: 623–627

Jones CL, Khan SA (1986) Nucleotide sequence of the enterotoxin B gene from *Staphylococcus aureus*. J Bacteriol 166: 29–33

Khan SA, Novick RP (1982) Structural analysis of plasmid pSN2 in *Staphylococcus aureus*: no involvement in enterotoxin B production. J Bacteriol 149: 642–649

Kreiswirth BN, Novick RP, Schlievert PM, Bergdoll MS (1982) Genetic studies on staphylococcal strains from patients with toxic-shock syndrome. Ann Intern Med 96: 974–977

Kreiswirth BN, Lofdahl S, Betley MJ, O'Reilly M, Schlievert PM, Bergdoll MS, Novick RP (1983) The toxic shock syndrome exotoxin structural gene is not detectably transmitted by a prophage. Nature 305: 709–712

Kreiswirth BN, Handley JP, Schlievert PM, Novick RP (1987a) Cloning and expression of streptococcal pyrogenic exotoxin A and staphylococcal toxic shock syndrome toxin-1 in *Bacillus subtilis*. Mol Gen Genet 208: 84–87

Kreiswirth BN, Schlievert PM, Novick RP (1987b) Evaluation of coagulase-negative staphylococci for ability to produce toxic shock syndrome toxin-1. J Clin Microbiol 25: 2028–2029

Kreiswirth BN, Projan SJ, Schlievert PM, Novick RP (1989) TSST-1 is encoded by a variable genetic element. Rev Infect Dis 11: S83–S89

Lee CY, Iandolo JJ (1986) Integration of staphylococcal phage L54a occurs by site-specific recombination: structural analysis of the attachment site. Proc Natl Acad Sci USA 83: 5474–5478

Lee CY, Schmidt JJ, Johnson-Winegar AD, Spero L, Iandolo JJ (1987) Sequence determination and comparison of the exfoliative toxin A and toxin B genes from *Staphylococcus aureus*. J Bacteriol 169: 3904–3909

Lofdahl S, Guss B, Uhlen M, Philipson L, Lindberg M (1983) Gene for staphylococcal protein A. Proc Natl Acad Sci USA 80: 697–701

Mallonee DH, Glatz BA, Pattee PA (1982) Chromosomal mapping of a gene affecting enterotoxin A production in *Staphylococcus aureus*. Appl Environ Microbiol 43: 397–402

McKane L, Ferretti JJ (1981) Phage-host interactions and the production of type A streptococcal exotoxin in group A streptococci. Infect Immun 34: 915–919

Murray NE, Barten PI, Murray K (1973) Restriction of bacteriophage by *Escherichia coli* K. J Mol Biol 81: 395–407

Musser JM, Schlievert PM, Chow AW, Ewan P, Kreiswirth BN, Novick RP, Rosdahl VT, Naidu AS, Witte W, Selander RK (1990) A single clone of *Staphylococcus aureus* causes the majority of cases of toxic shock syndrome. Proc Natl Acad Sci USA 87: 225–229

Nida SK, Ferretti JJ (1982) Phage influence on the synthesis of extracellular toxins in group A streptococci. Infect Immun 36: 745–750

Nida SK, Houston CW, Ferretti JJ (1979) Erythrogenic toxin production by group A streptococci. In: Parker MT (ed) Pathogenic streptococci. Reedbooks, Chertsey

Novick RP, Khan SA, Murphy E, Iordanescu I, Edelman J, Krolewski J, Rush M (1980) Hitchhiking transposons and other mobile genetic elements and site-specific recombination systems in staphylococci. Cold Spring Harbor Symp Quant Biol 45: 67–76

Okubo S, Yanagida T, Fujita DJ, Ohlsson-Wiilhelm BM (1972) The genetics of bacteriophage SPO1. Biken J 15: 81–97

O'Toole PW, Foster TJ (1987) Nucleotide sequence of the epidermolytic toxin A gene of *Staphylococcus aureus*. J Bacteriol 169: 3910–3915

Pattee PA, Glatz BA (1980) Identification of a chromosomal determinant of enterotoxin A production in *Staphylococcus aureus*. Appl Environ Microbiol 39: 186–193

Peng HL, Novick RP, Kreiswirth B, Kornblum J, Schlievert P (1988) Cloning, characterization, and sequencing of an accessory gene regulator (*agr*) in *Staphylococcus aureus*. J Bacteriol 170: 4365–4372

Ranelli DM, Jones CL, Johns MB, Mussey GJ, Khan SA (1985) Molecular cloning of staphylococcal enterotoxin B gene in *Escherichia coli* and *Staphylococcus aureus*. Proc Natl Acad Sci USA 82: 5850–5854

Recsei P, Kreiswirth B, O'Reilly M, Schlievert PM, Gruss A, Novick RP (1985) Regulation of exoprotein gene expression by *agr*. In: The staphylococci Zentralbl Bakteriol [Suppl] 14: 701–706

Recsei P, Kreiswirth B, O'Reilly M, Schlievert PM, Gruss A, Novick RP (1986) Regulation of exoprotein gene expression in *Staphylococcus aureus* by *agr*. Mol Gen Genet 202: 58–61

Schlievert PM, Blomster DA (1983) Production of staphylococcal pyrogenic exotoxin type C: influence of physical and chemical factors. J Infect Dis 147: 236–242

Schlievert PM, Kelly JA (1984) Clindamycin-induced suppression of toxic-shock syndrome-associated exotoxin production. J Infect Dis 149: 471

Schlievert PM, Shands KN, Dan BB, Schmid GP, Nishimura RD (1981) Identification and characterization of an exotoxin from *Staphylococcus aureus* associated with toxic shock syndrome. J Infect Dis 143: 509–516

Schmidt JJ, Spero L (1983) The complete amino acid sequence of staphylococcal enterotoxin C1. J Biol Chem 258: 6300–6306

Schutzer SE, Fischetti VA, Zabriskie JB (1983) Toxic shock syndrome and lysogeny in *Staphylococcus aureus*. Science 220: 316–318

Shafer WM, Iandolo JJ (1978a) Chromosomal locus for staphylococcal enterotoxin B. Infect Immun 20: 273–278

Shafer WM, Iandolo JJ (1978b) Staphylococcal enterotoxin A: a chromosomal gene product. Appl. Environ Microbiol 36: 389–391

Shafer WM, Iandolo JJ (1979) Genetics of staphylococcal enterotoxin B in methicillin-resistant isolates of *Staphylococcus aureus*. Infect Immun 25: 902–911

Shalita Z, Hertman I, Sarid S (1977) Isolation and characterization of a plasmid involved with enterotoxin B production in *Staphylococcus aureus*. J Bacteriol 129: 317–325

Shortle D (1983) A genetic system for analysis of staphylococcal nuclease. Gene 22: 181–189

Stevens DL, Tanner MH, Winship J, Swarts R, Reis KM, Schlievert PM, Kaplan E (1989) Severe group A streptococcal infections associated with a toxic shock-like syndrome and scarlet fever toxin A. N Engl J Med 321: 1–7

Warren R, Rogolsky M, Wiley BB, Glasgow LA (1975) Isolation of extrachromosomal deoxyribonucleic acid for exfoliative toxin production from phage group II *Staphylococcus aureus*. J Bacteriol 122: 99–105

Weeks CR, Ferretti JJ (1984) The gene for type A streptococcal exotoxin (erythrogenic toxin) is located in bacteriophage T12. Infect Immun 46: 531–536

Weeks CR, Ferretti JJ (1986) Nucleotide sequence of the type A streptococcal exotoxin (erythrogenic toxin) gene from *Streptococcus pyogenes* bacteriophage T12. Infect Immun 52: 144–150

Yu CE, Ferretti JJ (1989) Molecular epidemiologic analysis of the type A streptococcal exotoxin (erythrogenic toxin) gene (*speA*) in clinical *Streptococcus pyogenes* strains. Infect Immun 57: 3715–3719

Zabriskie JB (1964) The role of temperate bacteriophage in the production of erythrogenic toxin by group A streptococci. J Exp Med 119: 761–780

T Cell Recognition of Superantigens

T. Herrmann and H. R. MacDonald

1 Introduction

The specificity of the immune system is determined by antigen (Ag) receptors clonally expressed on T and B lymphocytes. These differ remarkably in their ligand specificity: While the Ag receptors of B lymphocytes (immunoglobulins, Ig) bind to soluble Ag, the T cell Ag receptors (TCR) recognize Ag presented by cells in conjunction with products of the polymorphic major histocompatibility complex class I and class II genes (MHC class I/II) (Davis and Bjorkman 1988; Marrack and Kappler 1987). The molecular basis of Ag presentation is the proteolysis of the Ag into small peptides which bind in a groove formed by the two most polymorphic domains of the MHC molecules ($\alpha1$ and 2 for MHC class I molecules, and $\alpha1$ and $\beta1$ for MHC class II molecules) (Bjorkman et al. 1987a, b; Brown et al. 1988). The TCR recognizes this MHC/peptide complex (Davis and Bjorkman 1988).

Ludwig Institute for Cancer Research, Lausanne Branch, 1066 Epalinges, Switzerland

Two isotypes of the TCR can be distinguished (α/β and γ/δ). The majority of T lymphocytes express α/β TCR and are specific for the complexes of antigen-derived peptides presented by MHC molecules (MHC/Ag). A minor portion of T lymphocytes express the γ/δ TCR. Their physiological role and specificity is poorly understood (RAULET 1989). Both isotypes of the TCR consist of the antigen-specific α/β or γ/δ heterodimer noncovalently linked to the nonpolymorphic, signal transducing, CD3 heterooligomer. The different TCR specificities for the MHC/Ag are created by the somatic recombination of a number of variable elements during T cell maturation in the thymus. The mouse genome contains about 100 V (variable) and 50 J (junction) elements for the α chain and 25 V, 12 J, and 2 D (diversity) elements for the β chain. Their random recombination and the random insertion of up to six nucleotides (N sequences) between the variable elements during recombination could theoretically lead to 10^{15} TCR specificities (DAVIS and BJORKMAN 1988). Modeling the variable part of the TCR after the crystal structure of Fab fragments of Ig predicts several complementarity determining regions (CDR), which might serve as contact points for TCR:MHC/Ag. The CDR 1 and 2 located on the V regions are predicted to interact preferentially with two α helices of the MHC molecules embedding the Ag peptide. The junctional region between VJ_α and VDJ_β forms a third CDR which might interact preferentially with the antigenic peptide itself (CHOTHIA et al. 1988; DAVIS and BJORKMAN 1988; CLAVERIE et al. 1989). The role of a hypothetical fourth CDR (CLAVERIE et al. 1989; KOURILSKY et al. 1989) located on the V region of the β chain will be discussed later.

During T cell development in the thymus, a selection of the randomly generated TCR specificities takes place. This selection leads to the generation of a mature repertoire of TCR recognizing preferentially foreign peptides bound to self MHC molecules, but not extrathymic self peptides (although a relatively high proportion of T cells show cross-reactivity with foreign MHC molecules). A popular view on this process is that low-affinity interaction of the TCR with self MHC molecules (or self MHC/peptide complexes) expressed on the thymic epithelium allows survival and further maturation of the thymocytes ("positive selection"), while a high-affinity interaction with self MHC (MHC/peptide complexes) expressed by cells of hematopoeitic origin stops further maturation and leads to clonal deletion by induction of programmed cell death (MARRACK and KAPPLER1987; VON BOEHMER 1986). T cells selected for recognition of MHC class I/Ag express the CD8 molecule, whereas T cells specific for MHC class II/Ag express CD4. These molecules facilitate the TCR MHC/Ag interaction, most likely by binding to nonpolymorphic residues of the MHC class I or II molecules. In mouse (and to a lesser extent in human) the division of T cells into MHC class I- or MHC class II-restricted cells correlates well with their functional division into precursors of cytolytic and helper T cells, respectively (SWAIN 1983).

Recently, another class of ligands interacting specifically with the TCR has been described. These so called "superantigens" (SAgs) are defined operationally by the T cell response they elicit (KAPPLER et al. 1988; MACDONALD et al. 1988a; WHITE et al. 1989; JANEWAY et al. 1989). Thus SAgs activate a much higher proportion of unprimed T cells than antigens do (1%–20%) and, more importantly, they activate nearly all T cells expressing a particular TCR V_β. Thus SAg specificities of a T cell clone can be predicted from its V_β usage. Another important feature of SAg is their exclusive presentation by MHC class II molecules.

2 Exogenous and Endogenous SAgs

2.1 Test Systems for SAgs

Two types of SAgs can be distinguished: (1) Endogenous SAgs (EndSAgs) are T cell stimulatory determinants expressed by some cell types. Up to now they have been identified only in mice. (2) Exogenous SAgs (ExSAgs) are produced by a variety of microorganisms. The following systems are commonly used to test compounds for superantigenic properties. (a) Stimulation of unprimed mature T lymphocytes and determination of the V_β usage of the stimulated T cells; (b) stimulation of a panel of T cell clones or hybridomas of defined V_β; (c) testing for clonal deletion during thymic development. (Note that clonal deletion of SAg-reactive cells can also be induced in neonatal mice by administering EndSAg-expressing cells or ExSAgs).

Not all SAgs have been defined by all three methods but, in general, deletion of SAg-reactive cells in the thymus seems to be the most sensitive method. A survey of currently defined SAg, their V_β specificities, and the methods by which they have been defined is given in Table 1.

2.2 Endogenous Superantigens

The first clear correlation between TCR V_β usage and specificity was found for V_β17a and reactivity to the I-E isotype of MHC class II (KAPPLER et al. 1987). In fact, as revealed later, the V_β17a TCR were not specific for the I-E molecules themselves but for an unknown tissue-specific (B cell) determinant recognized in conjunction with I-E (MARRACK and KAPPLER 1988). This turns out to be the case for other correlations of I-E specificity and V_β usage as well (Table 1). The first link between TCR V_β usage and specificity for an already defined T cell stimulating determinant was found for V_β6 and 8.1 and the a allele of the minor lymphocyte stimulatory locus 1 (Mls 1[a]).

The *minor lymphocyte stimulatory locus* (Mls) was originally discovered in mice as a genetic trait controlling a unidirectional mixed lymphocyte reaction (MLR) between MHC identical animals (FESTENSTEIN 1974). Originally it was thought to be one locus with several alleles, but it is now thought to consist of several genetic loci, each with a dominant stimulatory allele (designated a) and a recessive silent "null" allele (designated b) (for review see ABE and HODES 1989).

Table 1. Characteristics of the T cell response to endogenous superantigens

Endogenous superantigen	V_β usage	Presented by	Known polymorphism	Detected by		Thymic deletion
				MLR	T cell clones or hybridomas	
Mls 1[a]	6[1]	I-E > I-A	+	+	+	+
	7[2]	I-E > I-A	+	?	+	+
	8.1[3]	I-E > I-A	+	+	+	+
	9[4]	I-E > I-A	+	?	?	+
Mls 2[a]	3[5-7]	I-E > I-A	+	+	+	+
3[a]	3[5-7]	I-E > I-A	+	+	−	+
Unknown	5.1 + 5.2[8,9]	I-E	+	?	+	+
Unknown	11[8-12]	I-E	+	+	+	+
Unknown	12[8-12]	I-E	+	?	?	+
Unknown	16[8,13]	I-E	+	?	?	+
Unknown	17a[14,15]	I-E	−	−	+	+

Superscript numbers refer to following references: 1 (MacDonald et al. 1988a), 2 (Okada et al. 1990), 3 (Kappler et al. 1988), 4 (Happ et al. 1989), 5 (Pullen et al. 1988), 6 (Abe et al. 1988), 7 (Pullen et al. 1989a), 8 (Bill et al. 1988), 9 (Palmer et al. 1989), 10 (Tomonari and Lovering 1988), 11 (Bill et al. 1989), 12 (Vacchio et al. 1990), 13 (Singer et al. 1990), 14 (Kappler et al. 1987), 15 (Marrack and Kappler 1988)

The nomenclature for Mls varies in the literature. Mls 1^a corresponds to Mls^a, Mls 2/3^a to Mls^c, Mls^d to the coexpression of Mls 1^a and 2/3^a, and Mls^b designates expression of the b alleles of all Mls genes. Although the a alleles of Mls induce vigorous T cell proliferation and lymphokine production in vitro, they do not elicit transplant rejection or lethal graft vs host reactions. Also, no antisera against Mls determinants have been produced so far.

2.3 Exogenous Superantigens

In contrast to EndSAgs which are biochemically undefined, some ExSAgs are defined in biochemical and genetic terms (MARRACK and KAPPLER 1990). Among them are some of the most potent, naturally occurring, T cell stimulating agents, which act at subpicomolar concentrations. ExSAgs include proteins produced by organisms such as the gram-positive bacteria *Staphylococcus aureus* and *Streptococcus pyogenes* as well as by *Mycoplasma arthritidis* (MARRACK and KAPPLER 1990; TOMAI et al. 1990; COLE et al. 1990). The best characterized ExSAgs are the enterotoxins of *S. aureus* (SEs). Seven SEs (designated SEA, B, C1, C2, C3, D, and E) sharing variable degrees of sequence homology are known. They have apparent molecular weights (MW) between 24 and 30 kDa and a characteristic intrachain disulfide bridge located around the center of the molecule (MARRACK and KAPPLER 1990; IANDOLO 1989). This disulfide bridge is missing in toxic shock syndrome toxin-1 (TSST-1), a 22 kDa protein which shares some sequence homology with SEs but lacks their emetic properties (IANDOLO 1989). Another exotoxin of *S. aureus* exhibiting superantigenic properties is the exfoliative toxin A (MARRACK and KAPPLER 1990). *S. pyogenes* produces two types of biochemically unrelated SAgs, the pyrogenic exotoxin A, which has some sequence homology to the SEs (MARRACK and KAPPLER 1990; IMANISHI et al. 1990), and a 30 kDa peptide derived from the M type 5 protein (TOMAI et al. 1990). The SAg produced by *M. arthritidis* (MAM, mycloplasma arthritidis mitogen) is a biochemically ill-defined soluble protein which shows some V_β specificity in its T cell stimulating properties (COLE et al. 1990).

3 Presentation of SAgs

3.1 Presentation of EndSAgs

All SAgs characterized to date are presented by MHC class II-bearing cells. The first evidence for a role of MHC class II in presentation of EndSAgs comes from differences in the strength of Mls 1^a-dependent T cell stimulation found between different MHC class II alleles. All I-E-positive strain haplotypes present the Mls 1^a determinant very well, I-E-negative strains bearing I-A^{b,f,s,k,p} are of intermediate efficiency, and I-A^q presents marginally or not at all (ABE and HODES 1989; ANDERSON et al. 1989). The hierarchy between potent and weak Mls 1^a-presenting

MHC class II alleles can be detected in MLR in vitro and by the different extent of intrathymic deletion of Mls 1^a-reactive clones in vivo. The superiority of some MHC class II molecules in EndSAg presentation is most striking for the $V_\beta 5,11,12$, and 17a stimulating SAgs, which can only be presented by I-E-bearing cells (Table 1). In this context it is interesting that the DR_α chain can substitute for the I-E_α chain in the presentation of the $V_\beta 11$ and 17a stimulating EndSAgs (LAWRENCE et al. 1989). Another line of evidence for the crucial role of MHC class II molecules in Mls 1^a presentation is the inhibition of the T cell response to Mls 1^a by MHC class II specific monoclonal antibodies (mAb) (JANEWAY and KATZ 1985). In line with genetic experiments, the inhibitory capacity of I-E-specific mAb is greater than I-A-specific mAb, and combinations of mAb against both isotypes block a Mls-dependent MLR completely (although some authors report complete inhibition of Mls responses by I-E- or I-A-specific mAb alone) (WEBB and SPRENT 1989).

EndSAgs differ from conventional peptide Ags not only in being presented by a relatively large number of MHC class II alleles, but, more importantly, in their ability to be recognized even when presented by allogenic MHC molecules. This has been observed in MLRs in which responders and stimulators differ in both Mls and MHC alleles and in which the Mls 1^a-specific $V_\beta 6$ and $V_\beta 8.1$ T cells are preferentially stimulated (MACDONALD et al. 1990; LARSSON-SCIARD et al. 1990).

An important requirement for the presentation of protein antigens is their proteolytic fragmentation (antigen processing). It is not known whether this is also true for the presentation of EndSAgs. One interesting feature of Mls presentation is that any manipulation affecting the integrity of the membrane of the Mls-presenting cells, such as fixation with very low doses (0.1%) of paraformaldehyde, seems to functionally destroy the Mls 1^a determinant (unpublished observation). Interestingly, a negative correlation between the mobility of I-E molecules in the plasma membrane and the Mls 1^a allele has been reported, and it has been suggested that the composition of the membrane or interaction of MHC class II with membrane components could be critical for the presentation of EndSAg determinants (MECHERI et al. 1990a, b).

Not all MHC class II-bearing cells present EndSAg determinants, and the lack of specific reagents does not allow us to distinguish whether this is due to the lack of gene expression or to some special requirements for the expression of the superantigenic determinants at the cell surface. In vitro primary B cells and some B cell lines express superantigenic determinants but other professional antigen-presenting cells, e.g., macrophages and dendritic cells, do not (MOLINA et al. 1989; WEBB et al. 1989). This result is consistent with the presentation of Mls 1^a and other EndSAg determinants by radiosensitive hematopoeitic cells in vivo (MACDONALD et al. 1989; PULLEN et al. 1989b). An interesting aspect of the presentation of Mls 1^a by B cells is the activation of DNA synthesis and antibody production in Mls 1^a but not Mls 1^b B cells by mitomycin-treated, Mls 1^a-specific, helper clones (KATZ et al. 1986). Cognate T-B interaction has been observed in vitro for the ExSAg TSST-1 and MAM, but it is not clear whether this is also the case for the humoral immune response in vivo (MOURAD et al. 1989; TUMANG et al. 1990).

Finally, it should be mentioned that two recent reports have been interpreted as evidence for the expression of Mls 1[a] determinants on MHC class II-negative cells: (1) clonal deletion of Mls 1[a]-reactive T cells after neonatal injection of highly purified (presumably MHC class II-negative) CD8 T cells (WEBB and SPRENT 1990b); (2) skewing of the proportion of $V_\beta 6$ CD8 + T cells in an allo-H-2 MLR using purified Mls 1[a] ConA blast T cells as stimulators (LARSSON-SCIARD et al. 1990).

3.2 Presentation of ExSAgs

In contrast to the biochemically undefined EndSAgs, the presentation of ExSAgs is much better understood (Table 2). ExSAgs bind with relatively high affinity (K_d up to $10^{-8}\,M$) to MHC class II molecules on the cell surface or in detergent lysates (FISCHER et al. 1989; FRASER 1989; SCHOLL et al. 1989; HERRMANN et al. 1989; MOLLICK et al. 1989). T cell recognition of the ExSAg requires no processing, since SE and MAM can be presented by purified, immobilized, MHC class II molecules and by fixed antigen-presenting cells (BEKOFF et al. 1987; LEE and WATTS 1990). By contrast, proteolytic fragments of SEA do not stimulate T cells (FRASER 1989). Major differences between presentation of Ag and ExSAg have also been found using L cells transfected with I-A[k] variants. Substituting residues located in the hypothetical peptide binding site of I-A[k] by alanine dramatically affected the recognition of Ag (hen egg lysozyme peptide) but not of ExSAg (SEB). Conversely, mutating residues outside the putative peptide binding site

Table 2. V_β usage in the T cell response to exogenous superantigens

Exogenous superantigen	Human V_β	Mouse V_β
SEA	?	1, 3, 10, 11, 12, 17[1,5,6]
SEB	3, 12, 14, 15, 17, 20[1 3]	3[a], 7, 8.1–3, 17, 6[b1,6 9]
SEC1	12?[1,3]	3, 8.2, 8.3, 11, 17[1,6]
SEC2	12, 13.1, 13.2, 14, 15, 17, 20[1,3]	3, 8.2, 10, 17[1,6]
SEC3	5, 12, ?[1,3]	3, 7, 8.1, 8.2,[1,6]
SED	5, 12, ?[1,3]	3, 7, 8.1,–8.3, 11, 17[1,6]
SEE	5.1, 6.1–6.3, 8, 18[1 3]	11, 15, 17[1,6]
TSST-1	2[2,3]	3, 15, 17[1,6]
Exfoliative toxin A	2[2,3]	3, 10, 11, 15[1,6]
MAM	?	6, 8.1–8.3[10]
Streptococcus pyogenes		
Exotoxin A	?	8.2[11]
Pseudomonas aeruguenosa	?	
Exotoxin A		3, 5.1[12]
Type 5M protein	8, ?[4]	?

Superscript numbers refer to following references: 1 (MARRACK and KAPPLER 1990), 2 (KAPPLER et al. 1989), 3 (CHOI et al. 1989), 4 (TOMAI et al. 1990), 5 (TAKIMOTO et al. 1990), 6 (CALLAHAN et al. 1990), 7 (WHITE et al. 1989), 8 (JANEWAY et al. 1989), 9 (HERMAN et al. 1990), 10 (COLE et al. 1990), 11 (IMANISHI et al. 1990), 12 (MISFELDT 1990)
[a] Only at high concentrations
[b] If presented by human MHC class II+ cells (HERMAN et al. 1990)

diminished ExSAg but not Ag presentation (DELLABONA et al. 1990). Although not a direct proof, these findings fit with the concept that both ligands bind to different sites on the MHC class II molecule.

As for EndSAgs the efficiency of presentation of ExSAgs varies with MHC class II iso- and allotypes. The most striking example is MAM, which is presented only by I-E-bearing cells (COLE et al. 1981). These differences in recognition of ExSAgs reflect, at least partially, different MHC class II binding properties. For example, among the MHC class II molecules found in detergent extracts of the human B cell lymphoma RAJI, DR molecules bind most efficiently to SEA, and DQ to SEC1, 2, and 3, but all SE bind very weakly to DP (HERRMANN et al. 1989). In general, mouse MHC class II molecules bind and present SE weakly compared to human MHC class II molecules. This finding has been related to the fact that S. aureus is a common human but not mouse pathogen (MARRACK and KAPPLER 1990); however, this interpretation might go too far since TSST-1, a S. aureus product like the SE, binds to mouse and human MHC with similiar affinity (UCHIYAMA et al. 1989; SCHOLL et al. 1989). The weak response of mouse T cells to SE can be overcome by using human cells as presenting cells. This can lower the SE dose required for the half-maximal stimulation of T cell clones 100- to 1000-fold (HERRMANN et al. 1991) and leads to the detection of additional SE specificities (HERMAN et al. 1990).

MHC class II molecules present ExSAgs very efficiently, but it should be pointed out that cases of MHC class II-independent recognition of ExSAgs have been reported. First, induction of calcium influx of some Jurkat (human T leukemia) clones by both soluble SEA/SEB- and SEB-dependent proliferation of mouse T cell clones, in the absence of accessory cells, has been shown to occur (FLEISCHER and SCHREZENMEIER 1988; YAGI et al. 1990). Second, stimulation of human lymphocytes by (immobilized) streptococcal M type 5 protein in the presence of costimuli, e.g. PMA, was shown (KOTB et al. 1990). Finally, SE-dependent lysis of putatively MHC class II-negative cells by CD8 CTL clones has been demonstrated. The first two types of experiments have been interpreted as evidence for low-affinity binding of free ExSAg to the TCR. The SEB/SEC1-dependent cytolysis of MHC class II-negative cells could indicate the expression of an ExSAg-presenting molecule distinct from MHC class II (HERRMANN et al. 1991; DOHLSTEN et al. 1991).

4 T Cell Responses to SAgs

4.1 Both CD4 and CD8 T Cells Respond to SAgs Presented by MHC Class II

Control of SAg specificity by the V_β element of the TCR (KAYE and HEDRICK 1988) and inhibition studies with TCR-specific mAb provide evidence that MHC/Ag and SAg act via the TCR (KATZ and JANEWAY 1985). Now the question arises, are there qualitative differences or does the SAg act like a very strong Ag? The control of SAg specificity by the V_β element speaks against a mimicking of the Ag peptide by the SAg (although some T cell responses to Ag also show a remarkable limitation in V_β usage). If complexes of MHC class II and SAg would mimic complexes of MHC class II and peptide, one would expect the SAg-specific T cells to be MHC class II-restricted CD4 T cells. This is certainly not the case for ExSAgs and only to a limited extent for EndSAgs.

ExSAgs like SE and MAM, have been shown to activate both CD4 and CD8 cells in a MHC class II-dependent fashion (FLEISCHER and SCHREZENMEIER, 1988; MATTHES et al. 1988). A detailed study of the mouse T cell response to SEB (HERRMANN et al. 1990) showed that an equal proportion of $V_\beta 8$-bearing CD4 and CD8 T cells were stimulated. Furthermore, the SEB-primed CD8 T cells lysed MHC class II-bearing but not MHC class II-negative targets in a SEB-dependent manner. The same was observed for $V_\beta 8$-bearing CTL clones of defined Ag specificity and MHC class I restriction, which had not been previously exposed to SEB. The SEB-dependent cytotoxicity of these clones was MHC class II-dependent but independent of CD8 or of expression of MHC class I by the target cell.

These results appear to be in striking contrast to what is known about the T cell response to the EndSAg Mls 1[a]. Historically, this response has been considered to be limited to the CD4 T cell subset for a number of reasons: (1) CD4 but not CD8 cells are stimulated in a Mls-controlled primary MLR (JANEWAY et al. 1980); (2) the response of Mls-specific clones and hybridomas can be inhibited by CD4-specific mAb (KATZ and JANEWAY 1985); (3) only one CD8 CTL clone responding to Mls 1[a] has been reported (BRACIALE and BRACIALE 1981); (4) neonatal administration of CD4-specific mAb prevents clonal deletion of both CD4 and CD8 $V_\beta 6^+$ thymocytes in Mls 1[a] mice, suggesting that CD4 but not CD8 is necessary for recognition of Mls 1[a] by the immature CD4 and CD8 expressing thymocytes (MACDONALD et al. 1988c).

More recent experiments testing the IL-2 dependent expansion of $V_\beta 6$ and $V_\beta 8.1$ CD8$^+$ T cells after stimulation with Mls 1[a] B cells demonstrated that CD8 cells can recognize Mls 1[a], although to a lesser extent than CD4 T cells. Similar results were obtained in vivo after reconstitution of irradiated animals with Mls 1[a] stimulator cells (B cells) and Mls 1[b] responder cells (MACDONALD et al. 1990; WEBB and SPRENT 1990a). The reactivity of CD8 T cells to EndSAgs is not a peculiarity of the Mls 1a system since similar results have been obtained for the in vivo response of $V_\beta 11$ CD4 and CD8 T cells to an I-E dependent SAg. The analysis of thoracic duct lymphocytes after reconstitution of lethally irradiated I-E-positive mice ($V_\beta 11$ deleting) with lymphocytes of I-E-negative mice ($V_\beta 11$ nondeleting) showed, after the first day, a sharp decrease of $V_\beta 11$ CD4 and CD8 T cells (negative selection) but later on a high proportion of $V_\beta 11$ CD4 and CD8 T blasts (positive selection) (GAO et al. 1989). The question then arises, do CD8 T cells see Mls 1[a] in conjunction with MHC class II? They do, as demonstrated by comparison of Mls 1[a] presentation by different MHC class II haplotypes which affected the T cell response of CD4 and CD8 cells similiarly. Furthermore, MHC class II- but not MHC class I-specific mAb inhibited the activation of Mls 1[a]-reactive CD4 and CD8 T cells (CHVATCHKO and MACDONALD 1991). In all experiments the Mls 1[a] response of CD8 T cells appeared weaker than the response of CD4 T cells. Whether this apparently lower affinity of CD8 T cells for Mls 1[a] is due to the original selection of the TCR by MHC class I or the lack of CD4: class II MHC interaction is not clear. Such a low affinity might explain recently described differences in signals elicited by Ag and EndSAg. In these experiments only the recognition of MHC/Ag but not of Mls 1[a] activated inositol phosphate metabolism, although in both cases a strong proliferative response was observed (O'ROURKE et al. 1990). Whether this or other differences in signaling are related to the failure to detect Mls 1[a]-specific cytotoxicity of Mls 1[a]-primed CD8 T cells or CTL clones expressing the presumably Mls-reactive $V_\beta 6$ or 8.1 TCR remains to be elucidated (CHVATCHKO and MACDONALD, unpublished data).

4.2 Different Parts of the TCR are Required to Recognize Ags and SAgs

More precise information on the interaction of the TCR with MHC/SAg has been obtained by genetic manipulation of the TCR itself (PULLEN et al. 1990; CHOI et al. 1990). A first hint on residues possibly important for Mls 1[a] specificity came from the identification of the b and c alleles of $V_\beta 8.2$, which occur in some wild mice. About half of the $V_\beta 8.2^b$- and nearly all $V_\beta 8.2^c$-bearing T cells recognize Mls 1[a], but only very few T cells carrying the $V_\beta 8.2^a$ allele common to inbred strains. PULLEN et al. (1990) constructed T cell hybridomas expressing chimeric TCR, in which a $V_\beta 8.2^a$ domain was substituted with the residues found in $V_\beta 8.2^c$ at positions 22, 70, and 71 or all three. These hybridomas became Mls 1[a]-reactive without losing their Ag specificity. Residues in a similar region of the V_β domain were found to confer specificity for exotoxins. This was demonstrated for the SEC2 specificity by constructing hybridomas expressing chimeric V_β domains. The substitutions of residues 67–78 of SEC2 unreactive $V_\beta 13.1$ domain with those of the SEC2-reactive $V_\beta 13.2$ domain was sufficient to confer SEC2 reactivity (CHOI et al. 1990). Although mutational analysis by itself cannot answer the question whether these TCR residues actually bind to the ET/MHC class II complex, both the dissociation of EndSAg and Ag specificity and the important role of homologous regions for EndSAg and ExSAg specificity suggest a distinct TCR binding site for SAg. This site could be a fourth CDR, proposed by KOURILSKY et al. (1989) to be located in the V_β domain. In their model this CDR4 could interact with an altered conformation of the MHC class II molecule, but of course one could also imagine an interaction with a MHC class II-associated SAg molecule (CLAVERIE et al. 1989). In the context of these findings it would be interesting to see whether this putative fourth CDR would be also predicted for the γ chain of the TCR, since ExSAg-dependent lysis of MHC class II-bearing targets by $\gamma\delta$ cells (FLEISCHER and SCHREZENMEIER 1988; MATTHES et al. 1988) and a correlation between γ 9 usage and SEA reactivity have been reported (RUST et al. 1990).

5 Models of Mechanism of Action and Physiological Role of SAgs

5.1 Mechanism of Action of EndSAgs

The mechanism of T cell activation by EndSAgs will be discussed under the premise that: (a) MHC/Ag and EndSAgs bind to different sites on the same TCR (an alternative possibility, namely, the existence of a discrete Mls-1[a] receptor has been suggested based on segregation of MHC/Ag and Mls 1[a] specificities in T cell hybridomas and is discussed in WEBB and SPRENT, 1989) and (2) EndSAg recognition requires the presence of class II MHC molecules at the cell surface.

Taking Mls as a prototypic EndSAg, the following possibilities could be envisaged. First, Mls interacts directly with the TCR. The role of the MHC class II molecule would then be to position the Mls molecule such that it can interact effectively with the TCR. In this case the Mls molecule could be physically associated with MHC class II before it is recognized by the T cell but subsequent to a low-affinity interaction between the TCR and MHC class II. Second, the Mls determinant is directly recognized by the TCR but only after the Mls molecule has undergone a conformational change prompted by its binding to MHC class II. Third, the Mls determinant is induced on the MHC class II molecule as a consequence of the interaction of the MHC class II with a molecule under the control of the Mls locus. This induction could be due to a chemical modification but superantigenic conformations of MHC class II molecules could also be imagined. The possible Mls gene products inducing such a chemical modification or conformation could be MHC binding proteins or peptides but also enzymes or even lipids in the plasma membrane. We see at the moment no evidence in special favor of any model.

5.2 Mechanism of Action of ExSAgs

How do ExSAg function? We see three main possibilities: (1) ExSAgs bind directly to the TCR. Consequently, the only function of MHC molecules would be to immobilize them. This would explain why the correlation between V_β usage and specificity for a given ExSAg is relatively independent of iso-, allo-, or xenotype. Furthermore, the recognition of ExSAg on MHC class II-negative targets and proliferation in the absence of MHC class II-bearing cells, as has been observed in the presence of costimuli such as PMA, would be consistent with this model. In the latter instance one could imagine that the cell:cell interaction provides such a necessary costimulus. (2) The MHC class II molecule has a function beyond immobilizing the ExSAg. For example, the binding of the ExSAg to MHC class II may induce a TCR binding conformation of the ExSAg or, alternatively, the TCR may recognize epitopes on ExSAg and MHC class II at the same time. This model would explain those quantitative differences in ExSAg presentation by different MHC class II haplo- and isotypes which cannot be readily explained by differential binding (WHITE et al. 1989; SCHOLL et al. 1990; HERMANN et al. 1990). (3) By analogy with the arguments used for EndSAgs, the binding of ExSAg to MHC class II may induce the expression of V_β specific determinants on the MHC class II molecule. However, experiments demonstrating the complete loss of T cell activating properties by fragments of SEA that retain their MHC class II binding argue against the simplest version of this model (HERMANN and DOHLSTEN, unpublished data).

5.3 Do EndSAgs Act as Helper Determinants in Ag Recognition?

If it is true that a TCR has distinct MHC/peptide Ag and SAg binding sites, it is of interest to consider models of concomitant recognition of MHC/peptide Ag and EndSAg, either by different TCR on the same cells or by the same TCR molecule. In the first case the number of TCR molecules interacting with an antigen-presenting cell (i.e., avidity) would be increased, whereas in the second case the bivalency of the binding site would result in increased affinity of TCR/MHC interaction. Both situations would lead to a preferential activation of T cells expressing a V_β able to interact with an EndSAg. In such a model, in which the EndSAg functions as a helper determinant in T cell recognition, it would not be critical whether the SAg determinant is on the MHC molecule itself or is a MHC-associated molecule. In addition, it is theoretically possible that such SAg determinants enhancing the TCR/MHC Ag interaction are also MHC class I-associated but have not yet been detected, since their affinity for the TCR is too weak to trigger directly a T cell response. Such a concept of EndSAgs as helper molecules or determinants could help to explain the preferential usage of certain TCR V_β during positive selection in the thymus, where EndSAgs might facilitate the binding of TCR to self MHC molecules (MACDONALD et al. 1988b; ZUNIGA-PFLUCKER et al. 1989). TCR:EndSAg interaction could also increase the affinity of the TCR to complexes of MHC and foreign peptides and thus explain why in some immune responses a preferential usage of certain V_β has been observed. General theories of Mls as a helper or regulator in T cell activation have been formulated previously, but results of the experiments performed to test them have been contradictory (JANEWAY et al. 1983; HAMMERLING et al. 1988; NEEDLEMAN et al. 1988).

The above mentioned concept of EndSAgs as regulators of antigen recognition does not address the question of the physiological role of ExSAgs and their relationship to EndSAgs. This question is specifically addressed by the models discussed in the next section, but it could well be that there is no physiological link between EndSAgs and ExSAgs and that the only thing they have in common is their ability to stimulate T cells with high frequency. A polyclonal activation of lymphocytes could be beneficial for the microorganism since it could lead to suppression of the specific immune response (for review see REIMANN et al. 1990). In this regard the observation that ExSAgs bind to molecules involved in antigen recognition is not unusual, since binding of bacterial or viral products to MHC class I, MHC class II molecules, and different regions of Igs has been reported.

5.4 EndSAgs and the T Cell Repertoire

Aside from the idea of EndSAgs as regulators of the strength of antigen recognition, other models of the physiological function of EndSAgs have become quite popular. These latter models emphasize the ability of EndSAgs to shape the T cell repertoire by clonal deletion of EndSAg-specific cells and the cross-reactivity of T cells to EndSAgs and ExSAgs (KAPPLER et al. 1989). In fact, the number of V_β involved in the generation of the T cell repertoire in the mouse can be drastically reduced either by genetic mechanisms (i.e., deletion or mutation), which can neutralize up to 13 V_β elements, or by negative selection in the thymus, which (hypothesizing a mouse simultaneously expressing Mls 1[a], Mls 2/3[a], and the I-E-restricted EndSAg) could affect also up to 9 V_β elements. In evaluating the importance of such a dramatic reduction in the elements generating the T cell repertoire, one should keep in mind that the number of T cell specificities which can theoretically be generated with the remaining variable elements still exceeds the total number of T lymphocytes found in a mouse by several orders of magnitude. Furthermore, the widespread occurrence of deletion of V_β elements (due to genetic mechanisms or negative selection) among wild mice suggests that such events are of no major disadvantage to the immune system (PULLEN et al. 1988; KAPPLER et al. 1989a). The question is whether they are beneficial and two hypotheses have been made in support of this view. Common to both concepts is an advantage of EndSAgs over genomic deletion as a device to exclude V_β elements from the T cell repertoire, since expression of EndSAgs (as a genetically dominant trait) could efficiently reduce the phenoty-pic expression of certain V_β in a mouse population while maintaining the corresponding genes at high frequency. This would, in turn, allow rapid adaptation of the T cell repertoire to changing environmental conditions (PULLEN et al. 1988; KAPPLER et al. 1989a).

The first hypothesis on a positive effect of deletion of certain V_β elements by EndSAgs is based on studies of the V_β usage of autoimmune disease-inducing T cell clones. In the case of experimental allergic encephalitis, a preferential usage of $V_\beta 8.2$ (and $V_\alpha 4$) elements by pathogenic clones was reported and treatment of mice with $V_\beta 8$-specific mAb could cure the disease (ACHA-ORBEA et al. 1989; KUMAR et al. 1989). These findings strongly suggest that deletion of these V_β from the T cell repertoire by EndSAgs could reduce the risk of developing autoimmune diseases, but two questions remain to be answered. Is the preferential usage of these V_β really a peculiarity of autoimmune processes? Does clonal deletion of such T cells during generation of the T cell repertoire in the thymus prevent the generation of pathogenic clones using other V_β domains?

The second hypothesis suggests that deletion of V_β from the repertoire by EndSAgs is a mechanism to reduce the number of ExSAg-reactive cells (MARRACK and KAPPLER 1990). This hypothesis is supported by the fact that at least some of the pathophysiology of ExSAgs is linked to lymphokine production of T cells after stimulation with ExSAg and that in mice a direct correlation between the number of SEB-reactive T cells and weight loss after SEB administration has been found (MARRACK et al. 1990). However, one should mention that other pathological effects of staphylococcal exotoxins seem to be T cell-independent. For example, carboxymethylation of SEB destroys its emetic effect but not its T cell activating properties (ALBER et al. 1990). Also, the scalded skin syndrome caused by exfoliative toxin is unlikely to be a consequence of T cell activation since it can occur neonatally (MELISH and GLASGOW 1970; IANDOLO 1989).

Since both hypotheses are based on the observation that polymorphic EndSAgs shape the T cell repertoire in mice, it would be important to know whether this is true for other species as well. At present no such evidence has been found, possibly due to the following reasons: (1) Only very few V_β-specific mAb are available for the human system and rat. (2) The EndSAgs show little or no polymorphism, or the polymorphism is difficult to detect since many EndSAgs distributed in the population with high frequency could delete the same V_β. The latter situation would lead to a functional lack of polymorphism. In both cases the negative selection of certain V_β (occurring only in the thymus) would not be detected by comparing the peripheral T cell repertoire of different individuals. (3) EndSAgs as defined by their ability to stimulate a high proportion of T cells expressing a certain V_β element (or to delete thymocytes expressing certain V_β), only exist in mice. In this case they could still exist in other species in a weaker form and regulate T cell activation.

Note added in proof. Evidence for EndSAg being encoded by an open reading frame in the 3′ long terminal repeat of mouse mammary tumor virus has been provided. CHOI et al. (1991) Nature 350: 203–207. ACHA-ORBEA et al. (1991) Nature 350: 207–211.

References

Abe R, Hodes RJ (1989) T-cell recognition of minor lymphocyte stimulating (mls) gene products. Annu Rev Immunol 7: 683–708
Abe R, Vacchio MS, Fox B, Hodes RJ (1988) Preferential expression of the T-cell receptor V_β3 gene by Mls^c reactive T cells. Nature 335: 827–830
Acha-Orbea H, Steinman L, McDevitt HO (1989) T cell receptors in murine autoimmune diseases. Annu Rev Immunol 7: 371–405
Alber G, Hammer DK, Fleischer B (1990) Relationship between enterotoxic-and T lymphocyte-stimulating activity of staphylococcal enterotoxin B. J Immunol 144: 4501–4506
Anderson GD, Banerjee S, David CS (1989) MHC class II A$_z$ and E$_z$ molecules determine the clonal deletion of V_β6 cells. J Immunol 143: 3757–3761
Bekoff MC, Cole BC, Grey HM (1987) Studies on the mechanism of stimulation of T cells by the mycoplasma arthritidis-derived mitogen. J Immunol 139: 3189–3194
Bill J, Appel VB, Palmer E (1988) An analysis of T-cell receptor variable region gene expression in major histocompatibility complex disparate mice. Proc Natl Acad Sci USA 85: 9184–9188

Bill J, Kanagawa O, Woodland DL, Palmer E (1989) The MHC molecule I-E is necessary but not sufficient for the clonal deletion of V_β 11-bearing T cells. J Exp Med 169: 1405–1419

Bjorkman PJ, Saper MA, Samraoui B, Bennett WS, Strominger JL, Wiley DC (1987a) Structure of the human class I histocompatibility antigen, HLA-2. Nature 329: 506–512

Bjorkman PJ, Saper MA, Samraoui B, Bennett WS, Strominger JL, Wiley DC (1987b) The foreign antigen binding site and T cell recognition regions of class I histocompatibility antigens. Nature 329: 512–518

Braciale VL, Braciale TJ (1981) Mls locus recognition by a cloned line of H-2 restricted influenza virus-specific cytotoxic T lymphocytes. J Immunol 127: 859–862

Brown JH, Jardetzky T, Saper MA, Samraoui B, Bjorkman PJ, Wiley DC (1988) A hypothetical model of the foreign antigen binding site of class II histocompatibility molecules. Nature 332: 845–850

Callahan JE, Herman A, Kappler JW, Marrack P (1990) Stimulation of B10.BR T cells with superantigenic staphyloccal toxins. J Immunol 144: 2473–2479

Choi Y, Kotzin B, Herron L, Callahan J, Marrack P, Kappler J (1989) Interaction of staphylococcus aureus toxin "superantigens" with human T cells. Proc Natl Acad Sci USA 86: 8941–8945

Choi Y, Herman A, DiGiusto D, Wade T, Marrack P, Kappler J (1990) Residues of the variable region of the T-cell-receptor β-chain that interact with S. aureus toxin superantigens. Nature 346: 471–473

Chothia C, Boswell DR, Lesk AM (1988) The outline structure of the T-cell $\alpha\beta$ receptor. EMBO J 7: 3745–3755

Chvatchko Y, MacDonald HR (1991) CD8$^+$ T cell response to Mls 1^a determinants involves MHC class II molecules. J Exp Med 173: 779–782

Claverie J-M, Prochnika-Chalufour A, Bougueleret L (1989) Implications of a Fab-like structure for the T-cell receptor. Immunol Today 10: 10–14

Cole BC, Daynes RA, Ward JR (1981) Stimulation of mouse lymphocytes by a mitogen derived from mycoplasma arthritidis. I. Transformation is associated with an H-2-linked gene that maps to the I-E/I-C subregion. J Immunol 127: 1931–1936

Cole BC, Kartchner DR, Wells DJ (1990) Stimulation of mouse lymphocytes by a mitogen derived from mycoplasma arthritidis (MAM). VIII. Selective activation of T cells expressing distinct V_β T cell receptors from various strains of mice by the "superantigen" MAM. J Immunol 144: 425–431

Davis MM, Bjorkman PJ (1988) T-cell antigen receptor genes and T-cell recognition. Nature 334: 395–402

Dellabona P, Peccoud J, Kappler J, Marrack P, Benoist C, Mathis D (1990) Superantigens interact with MHC class II molecules outside the binding groove. Cell 62: 1115–1121

Dohlsten M, Hedlund G, Segren S, Lando PA, Herrmann T, Kelly AP, Kalland T (1991) Human MHC class II-colon carcinoma cells present staphyloccal superantigens to cytotoxic T lymphocytes: evidence for a novel enterotoxin receptor. Eur J Immunol 21: 1229–1233

Festenstein H (1974) Pertinent features of M locus determinants including revised nomenclature and strain distribution. Transplantation 18: 555–557

Fischer H, Dohlsten M, Lindvall M, Sjögren H-O, Carlsson R (1989) Binding of staphylococcal enterotoxin A to HLA-DR on B cell lines. J Immunol 142: 3151–3157

Fleischer B, Schrezenmeier H (1988) T cell stimulation by staphyloccal enterotoxins. Clonally variable response and requirement for major histocompatibility complex class II molecules on accessory or target cells. J Exp Med 167: 1697–1707

Fraser JD (1989) High affinity binding of staphylococcal enterotoxins A and B to HLA-DR. Nature 339: 221–223

Gao EK, Kanagawa O, Sprent J (1989) Capacity of unprimed CD4$^+$ and CD8$^+$ T cells expressing V_β11 receptors to respond to I-E alloantigens in vivo. J Exp Med 170: 1947–1957

Hämmerling U, Toulon M, Chun M, Palfree S, Hoffmann MK (1988) Bidirectionality of mixed lymphocyte stimulation (mls) response. Effects of mls^b stimulator cells on mls^a helper cells. J Immunol 140: 2543–2548

Happ MP, Woodland DL, Palmer E (1989) A third T-cell receptor β-chain variable region gene encodes reactivity to Mls-1^a gene products. Proc Natl Acad Sci USA 86: 6283–6396

Herman A, Croteau G, Sekaly R-P, Kappler J, Marrack P (1990) HLA-DR alleles differ in their ability to present staphylococcal enterotoxins to T cells. J Exp Med 172: 709–717

Herrmann T, Accolla RS, MacDonald HR (1989) Different staphyloccocal enterotoxins bind preferentially to distinct major histocompatibility complex class II isotypes. Eur J Immunol 19: 2171–2174

Herrmann T, Maryanski JL, Romero P, Fleischer B, MacDonald HR (1990) Activation of MHC class I-restricted CD8$^+$ CTL by microbial T cell mitogens. Dependence upon MHC class II expression of the target cells and V_β usage of the responder T cells. J Immunol 144: 1181–1186

Herrmann T, Romero P, Sartoris S, Paiola F, Accolla RS, Maryanski JL, MacDonald HR (1991) Staphylococcal enterotoxin-dependent lysis of MHC class II negative target cells by cytolytic T lymphocytes. J Immunol 146: 2504–2512

Iandolo JI (1989) Genetic analysis of extracellular toxins of *Staphylococcus aureus*. Annu Rev Microbiol 43: 375–402

Imanishi K, Igarashi H, Uchiyama T (1990) Activation of murine T cells by streptococcal pyrogenic exotoxin A. Requirement for MHC class II molecules on accessory cells and identification of V_β elements in T cell receptor of toxin-reactive T cells. J Immunol 14: 3170–3175

Janeway CA Jr, Katz ME (1985) The immunobiology of the T cell response to mls-locus-disparate stimulator cells. I. Unidirectionality, new strain combinations, and the role of Ia antigens. J Immunol 134: 2057–2063

Janeway CA Jr, Lerner EA, Jason JM, Jones B (1980) T lymphocytes responding to mls-locus antigens are lyt-1[+], 2- and I-A restricted. Immunogenetics 10: 481–497

Janeway CA Jr, Conrad PJ, Tite J, Jones B, Murphy DB (1983) Efficiency of antigen presentation differs in mice differing at the Mls locus. Nature 306: 80–83

Janeway CA Jr, Yagi J, Conrad PJ, Katz ME, Vroegop S, Buxser S (1989) T-cell responses to mls and to bacterial proteins that mimic its behavior. Immunol Rev 107: 61–88

Kappler J, Kotzin B, Herron L, Gelfand EW, Bigler RD, Boylston A, Carrel S, Posnett DN, Choi Y, Marrack P (1989) V_β-specific stimulation of human T cells by staphylococcal toxins. Science 244: 811–813

Kappler JW, Wade T, White J, Kushner E, Blackman M, Bill J, Roehm N, Marrack P (1987) A T cell receptor V_β segment that imparts reactivity to a class II major histocompatibility complex product. Cell 49: 262–271

Kappler JW, Staerz U, White J, Marrack P (1988) Self tolerance eliminates T cells specific for Mls-modified products of the major histocompatibility complex. Nature 332: 35–40

Kappler JW, Pullen A, Callahan J, Choi Y, Herman A, White J, Wakeland E, Marrack P (1989a) Consequence of self and foreign superantigen interaction with specific V_β elements of the murine TCR $\alpha\beta$. Cold Spring Harbor Symp Quant Biol 54: 401–407

Katz ME, Janeway CA Jr (1985) The immunobiology of T cell responses to mls-locus-disparate stimulator cells. II. Effects of mls-locus-disparate stimulator cells on cloned, protein antigen-specific, Ia restricted T cell lines. J Immunol 134: 2064–2078

Katz ME, Todd JK, Janeway CA Jr (1986) The immunobiology of T cell responses to Mls-locus-disparate stimulator cells. III. Helper and cytolytic functions of cloned, Mls-reactive T cell lines. J Immunol 136: 1–5

Kaye J, Hedrick SM (1988) Analysis of specificity for antigen, Mls, and allogeneic MHC by transfer of T-cell receptor α-and β-chain genes. Nature 336: 580–583

Kotb M, Majumdjar G, Tomai M, Beachy EH (1990) Accessory cell-independent stimulation of human T cells by streptococcal M protein superantigen. J Immunol 145: 1332–1336

Kourilsky P, Claverie J-M, Prochnicka-Chalufour A, Spetz-Hagberg A-L, Larsson-Sciard E-L (1989) How important is the direct recognition of polymorphic MHC residues by TCR in the generation of the T-cell repertoire. Cold Spring Harbor Symp Quant Biol 54: 93–103

Kumar V, Kono DH, Urban JL, Hood L (1989) The T-cell receptor repertoire and autoimmune diseases. Annu Rev Immunol 7: 657–682

Larsson-Sciard E-L, Spetz-Hagberg A-L, Casrouge A, Kourilsky (1990) Analysis of T cell receptor V_β gene usage in primary mixed lymphocyte reactions: evidence for directive usage by different antigen-presenting cells and mls-like determinants on T cell blasts. Eur J Immunol 20: 1223–1229

Lawrance SK, Karlsson L, Price J, Quaranta V, Yacov R, Sprent J, Petterson PA (1989) Transgenic HLA-DR$_\alpha$ faithfully reconstitutes IE-controlled immune functions and induces cross-tolerance to E_α E_α0 mutant mice. Cell 58: 583–594

Lee JM, Watts TH (1990) Binding of staphyloccocal enterotoxin A to purified murine MHC class II molecules in supported lipid bilayers. J Immunol 144: 3360–3366

MacDonald HR, Schneider R, Lees RK, Howe RC, Acha-Orbea H, Festenstein H, Zinkernagel RM, Hengartner H (1988a) T-cell receptor V_β use predicts reactivity and tolerance to Mls[a]-encoded antigens. Nature 332: 40–45

MacDonald HR, Lees RK, Schneider R, Zinkernagel RM, Hengartner H (1988b) Positive selection of CD4[+] thymocytes controlled by MHC class II gene products. Nature 336: 471–473

MacDonald HR, Hengartner H, Pedrazzini T (1988c) Intrathymic deletion of self reactive cells prevented by anti-CD4 antibody treatment. Nature 335: 174–176

MacDonald HR, Glasebrook AL, Schneider R, Lees RK, Pircher H, Pedrazzini T, Kanagawa O, Nicolas J-F, Howe RC, Zinkernagel RM, Hengartner H (1989) T-cell reactivity and tolerance to Mls[a]-encoded antigens. Immunol Rev 107: 89–108

MacDonald HR, Lees RL. Chvatchko Y (1990) CD8[+] T cells respond clonally to Mls-1[a]-encoded determinants. J Exp Med 171: 1381–1386

Marrack P, Kappler J (1987) The T cell receptor. Science 238: 1073–1079

Marrack P, Kappler J (1988) T cells distinguish between allogeneic major histocompatibility complex products on different cell types. Nature 332: 840–842

Marrack P, Kappler J (1990) The staphylococcal enterotoxins and their relatives. Science 248: 705–711

Marrack P, Blackman M, Kushnir E, Kappler J (1990) The toxicity of staphylococcal enterotoxin B in mice is mediated by T cells. J Exp Med 171: 455–464

Matthes M, Schrezenmeier H, Homfeld J, Fleischer S, Malissen B, Kirchner H, Fleischer B (1988) Clonal analysis of human T cell activation by the mycoplasma arthritidis mitogen (MAS). Eur J Immunol 18: 1733–1737

Mecheri S, Edidin M, Dannecker G, Mittler RS, Hoffmann MK (1990a) Immunogenic Ia-binding peptides immobilize the Ia molecule and facilitate its aggregation on the B cell membrane. Control by the mls-1 gene. J Immunol 144: 1361–1368

Mecheri S, Dannecker G, Dennig D, Hoffmann MK (1990b) Immunogenic peptides require an undisturbed phospholipid cell membrane environment and must be amphipatic to immobilize Ia on B cells. J Immunol 144: 1369–1374

Melish ME, Glasgow LA (1970) The staphylococcal scalded skin syndrome. Development of an experimental model. N Engl J Med 282: 1114–1119

Misfeldt ML (1990) Microbial "superantigens". Infect Immun 58: 2409–2413

Molina IJ, Cannon NA, Hyman R, Huber BT (1989) Macrophages and T cells do not express Mls[a] determinants. J Immunol 143: 39–44

Mollick JA, Cook RG, Rich RR (1989) Class II MHC molecules are specific receptors for staphylococcus enterotoxin A. Science 244: 817–821

Mourad W, Scholl P, Diaz A, Geha R, Chatila T (1989) The staphyloccal toxic shock syndrome toxin 1 triggers B cell proliferation via major histocompatibility complex-unrestricted cognate T/B cell interaction. J Exp Med 170: 2011–2023

Needleman BW, Lynch DH, Hodes RJ (1988) Effect of Mls 1[a] on antigen presentation to class II-restricted T cells. J Immunol 141: 3760–3767

Okada CY, Holzmann B, Guidos C, Palmer E, Weissmann IL (1990) Characterisation of a rat monoclonal antibody specific for a determinant encoded by the $V_\beta 7$ gene segment. J Immunol 144: 3473–3477

O'Rourke AM, Mescher MF, Webb SR (1990) Activation of polyphosphoinsositide hydrolysis in T cells by H-2 alloantigen but not mls determinants. Science 249: 171–174

Palmer E, Woodland DL, Happ MP, Bill J, Kanagawa O (1989) A third set of genes that regulates thymic selection. Cold Spring Harbor Symp Quant Biol 54: 135–145

Pullen AM, Marrack P, Kappler JW (1988) The T-cell repertoire is heavily influenced by tolerance to polymorphic self-antigens. Nature 335: 796–801

Pullen AM, Marrack P, Kappler JW (1989a) Evidence that Mls-2 antigens which delete $V_\beta 3^+$ T cells are controlled by multiple genes. J Immunol 142: 3033–3037

Pullen AM, Kappler JW, Marrack P (1989b) Tolerance to self antigens shapes the T-cell repertoire. Immunol Rev 107: 125–140

Pullen AM, Wade T, Marrack P, Kappler JW (1990) Identification of the region of T cell receptor $\bar\beta$ chain that interacts with the self-superantigen mls-1[a]. Cell 29: 1365–1374

Raulet DH (1989) The structure, function, and molecular genetics of the γ/δ T cell receptor. Annu Rev Immunol 7: 175–207

Reimann J, Claesson MH, Qvirin N (1990) Suppression of the immune response by microorganisms. The paradox: interactions of bacteria with invariant (monomorphic) determinants of antigen receptors and MHC molecules. Scand J Immunol 31: 543–546

Ruşt CJJ, Verreck F, Vietor H, Koning F (1990) Specific recognition of staphylococcal enterotoxin A by human T cells bearing receptors with the $V_\gamma 9$ region. Nature 346: 572–574

Scholl PR, Diez A, Mourad W, Parsonett J, Geha RS, Chatila T (1989) Toxic shock syndrome toxin 1 binds to major histocompatibility complex class II molecules. Proc Natl Acad Sci USA 86: 4210–4214

Scholl PR, Diez A, Karr R, Sekaly R-P, Trowsdale J, Geha R (1990) Effect of isotypes and allelic polymorphism on the binding of staphylococcal exotoxins to MHC class II molecules. J Immunol 144: 226–230

Singer PA, Balderas RS, Theofilopoulos AN (1990) Thymic selection defines multiple T cell receptor V_β "repertoire phenotypes" at the CD4/CD8 subset level. EMBO J 9: 3641–3648

Swain SL (1983) T cell subsets and the recognition of MHC class. Immunol Rev 74: 129–142

Takimoto H, Yoshikai Y, Kishihara K, Matsuzaki M, Kuga H, Otani T, Nomoto K (1990) Stimulation of all T cells bearing $V_\beta 1$, $V_\beta 3$, $V_\beta 11$, $V_\beta 12$ by staphylococcal enterotoxin A. Eur J Immunol 20: 617–621

Tomai M, Kotb M, Majumdjar G, Beachey EH (1990) Superantigenicity of Streptococcal M protein. J Exp Med 172: 359–362

Tomonari K, Lovering E (1988) T cell receptor-specific monoclonal antibodies against a $V_\beta 11$-positive mouse T-cell clone. Immunogenetics 28: 445–451

Tumang JR, Posnett DN, Cole BC, Crow MK, Friedman SM (1990) Helper T cell-dependent human B cell differentiation mediated by mycoplasmal superantigen bridge. J Exp Med 171: 2153–2158

Uchiyama T, Tadakuma T, Imanishi K, Araake A, Saito S, Yan X-J, Fujikawa H, Igarashi H, Yamaurea N (1989) Activation of murine T cells by toxic shock syndrome toxin-1. The toxin-binding structures expressed on murine accessory cells are MHC class II molecules. J Immunol 143: 3175–3182

Vacchio MS, Ryan JJ, Hodes RJ (1990) Characterisation of the ligand(s) responsible for negative selection of $V_\beta 11$- and $V_\beta 12$-expressing T cells: effects of a new mls determinant. J Exp Med 172: 807–813

Von Boehmer H (1986) The selection of the α, β heterodimeric T-cell receptor for antigen. Immunol Today 7: 333–336

Webb SR, Sprent J (1989) T-cell responses and tolerance to Mls[a] determinants. Immunol Rev 107: 141–158

Webb SR, Sprent J (1990a) Response of mature unprimed CD8[+] T cells to Mls[a] determinants. J Exp Med 171: 953–958

Webb SR, Sprent J (1990b) Induction of neonatal tolerance to Mls[a] antigens by CD8[+] T cells. Science 248: 1643–1646

Webb SR, Okamoto A, Ron Y, Sprent J (1989) Restricted tissue distribution of mls 1[a] determinants. Stimulation of mls 1[a]-reactive T cells by B cells but not by dendritic cells or macrophages. J Exp Med 169: 1–12

White J, Herman A, Pullen AM, Kubo R, Kappler JW, Marrack P (1989) The V_β-specific superantigen staphylococcal enterotoxin B: stimulation of mature T cells and clonal deletion in neonatal mice. Cell 56: 27–35

Yagi J, Baron J, Buxser S, Janeway CA Jr (1990) Bacterial proteins that mediate the association of a defined subset of T cell receptor: CD4 complexes with class II MHC. J Immunol 144: 892–901

Zuniga-Pflucker JC, Longo DL, Kruisbeek AM (1989) Positive selection of CD4-CD8[+] T cells in the thymus of normal mice. Nature 338: 76–78

T Cell Activation by Superantigens—
Dependence on MHC Class II Molecules

H. O. SJÖGREN

1 Introduction

The capacity of certain bacterial exoproducts to act as T cell mitogens has long been recognized (PEARY et al. 1970). Similar to other, polyclonal activators, they were found to require the participation of accessory cells (AC). It was later shown that the function of a cell type as AC correlated with its expression of MHC class II (CARLSSON et al. 1988; FLEISCHER and SCHREZENMEIER 1988). The number of microbial exoproducts shown to act as T cell mitogens in this way has gradually increased and these molecules have been called "superantigens" (SAs) in view of their capacity to activate a large proportion of all T lymphocytes in various species (MARRACK and KAPPLER 1990). The activation is induced by selective interaction with all T cells expressing certain V-β and V-γ chains of the T cell receptor (TCR) regardless of their epitope specificity. Besides other microbial molecules such as the *Mycoplasma arthritidis* protein MAM (COLE et al. 1981), this group of SAs also includes certain self molecules, the murine Mls antigens (JANEWAY 1990). There are strong indications that the Mls antigens are encoded by retroviral genes (MARRACK et al. 1991; FRANKEL et al. 1991; WOODLAND et al. 1991; DYSON et al. 1991). A dependence on class II-expressing AC has been

Department of Tumor Immunology, The Wallenberg Laboratory, University of Lund, 22007 Lund, Sweden demonstrated for all SAs studied, although at least for some SAs it can be replaced by a combination of other accessory signals. Besides their TCR binding and massive T cell activating capacity, this usage of MHC class II molecules is the most prominent common feature of SAs. With few exceptions this binding to MHC class II is a prerequisite for the T cell activating effects of SAs and is therefore of prime importance in their function.

2 SAs Bind with High Affinity to MHC Class II but not to Class I Molecules

Although SAs, even in minute quantities, are potent activators of T cells, their binding to T cells is usually not possible to demonstrate in direct binding assays. This finding is consistent with their failure to induce a proliferative response in resting T cells in the absence of AC, even in the presence of exogenous interleukin-1 (IL-1) and IL-2 (CARLSSON et al. 1988). In contrast, SAs bind to various AC, i.e., monocytes, B lymphocytes, and various B cell lines. A common important feature of all these cells is their expression of MHC class II molecules, which became evident when it was demonstrated that two monocytic cell lines, U937 and THP-1, that lack MHC class II expression also failed to bind staphylococcal enterotoxin A (SEA) and to function as AC in SEA-induced T cell activation, although they supported PHA-induced polyclonal activation (CARLSSON et al. 1988). The fact that Daudi cells, which lack expression of MHC class I molecules, bind staphylococcal enterotoxins (SEs) and support T cell activation very well (CARLSSON et al. 1988; FRASER 1989) rules out involvement of MHC class I molecules of AC in T cell activation in general and in activation of CD8$^+$ T cells in particular.

Electrophoresis of detergent extracts of the Raji B cell line demonstrated a distinct 60 kDa HLA-DR band which bound SEA (FISCHER et al. 1989). It was also shown that certain monoclonal antibodies (mAb) to HLA-DR could block the SEA binding to AC and the induction of T cell proliferation. Immunoprecipitation with mAb against HLA-DR and HLA-DQ showed that SEA bound to HLA-DR but failed to demonstrate DQ binding. Binding of labeled SEA to the Raji cell surface, followed by cross-linking and detergent solubilization of the cell membranes, electrophoresis, and western blotting, yielded two SEA-containing bands corresponding to Mr 90 and 105, which both also bound anti-DR mAb. This established that the major SEA binding molecule on Raji cells is HLA-DR, indicating that the binding of SEA to Raji cells with a K_a of approximately $1 \times 10^7 M^{-1}$ represents binding to HLA-DR expressed by these cells. Similarly, certain antibodies to HLA class II molecules and/or HLA-DR have been shown to block human T cell activation with other SAs (FLEISCHER and SCHEREZENMEIER 1988; SCHOLL et al. 1989).

The involvement of MHC class II molecules in SA-induced T cell activation is also evident from the finding that MHC class II-negative mutants of the Raji B cell line lack SE binding capacity and do not function as AC (MOLLICK et al. 1989). Further direct proof for the involvement of HLA class II molecules in the binding of SE leading to T cell activation comes from the demonstration that transfection of HLA-DR into fibroblasts (lacking capacity to bind SE) makes them capable of binding SEA and of supporting T cell activation (MOLLICK et al. 1989; SCHOLL et al. 1990a). Similar findings showing that SAs bind to MHC class II molecules, have been obtained in murine systems (COLE et al. 1990a; IMANISHI et al. 1990). The demonstration that T cells and T cell hybridomas can be activated by exposure to SA on purified I-E molecules inserted in lipid bilayers shows that MHC class II molecules are not only required but that they are also sufficient for T cell activation (LEE and WATTS 1990), although other molecules can indeed enhance the response (FLEISCHER et al. 1991; FISCHER et al. 1991).

Studies of T cell clones have shown that a given clone, irrespective of its antigen specificity and MHC restriction, can respond to SE in the presence of allogeneic AC (FLEISCHER and SCHEREZENMEIER 1988), which demonstrates that there is no restriction of the response by polymorphic portions of the class II molecules.

Not only $CD4^+$ but also $CD8^+$ T cells and $\gamma\delta$ TCR-bearing $CD4^-$ $CD8^-$ T cells respond to SE presented on the MHC class II of AC (FLEISCHER and SCHREZENMEIER 1988; FISCHER et al. 1990). However, there are indications of a low-affinity binding of SE directly to TCR that is not sufficient to elicit a full response of the T cells but which results in a rise of the cytosolic calcium concentration (FLEISCHER et al. 1988). $CD8^+$ cells become cytolytic when activated by SE with strict specificity for MHC class II-expressing target cells carrying SE (FLEISCHER and SCHREZENMEIER 1988; HEDLUND et al. 1990; HERRMANN et al. 1990). The role of the MHC class II molecule in T cell activation appears to be to enhance CD3 clustering by providing a multivalent SE and possibly to alter the SE conformation to increase the affinity to the V_β of TCR. With few exceptions the creation of multivalent SE by immobilization on plastic has not led to a strong activation of resting T cells in the absence of AC, which would tend to indicate the importance of a change in the appearance of SE when it is bound to MHC class II. SEs have also been shown to induce monocytes/macrophages to produce tumor necrosis factor-α (TNF-α) and IL-1 (JUPIN et al. 1988; FISCHER et al. 1990; GJÖRLOFF et al. 1991). Similar to the SE-induced T cell activation, TNF-α and IL-1 production appears to require binding of the SE to MHC class II molecules on the producing cells (MOLLICK et al. 1990) and, at least with some SEs, T cells must also be present (FISCHER et al. 1990; GJÖRLOFF et al. 1991). Preexposure of the monocytes to interferon-γ (IFN-γ) increases MHC class II expression, and this is presumed to explain the increased TNF production in response to toxic shock syndrome toxin-1 (TSST-1) recorded after IFN exposure (GROSSMAN et al. 1990). The role of T cells in TNF production by monocytes has not yet been clarified. It has been established that whereas purified $CD4^+ 45RO^+$ memory T cells supported TNF-α and II-1 production by purified monocytes, the presence of $CD4^+ 45RA^+$ naive helper and $CD8^+$ T cells did not (FISCHER et al. 1990; GJÖRLOFF et al. 1991). $CD4^+ 45RO^+$ memory T cells are also the main producers of IFN-γ, whereas the other two subpopulations produce only very small quantities. Thus this finding is consistent with the contention that the stimulatory effect on TNF production is mediated by IFN-γ (GROSSMAN et al. 1990). However, the participation of T cells in the production of TNF and IL-1 by monocytes could not be replaced by various T cell-derived recombinant lymphokines, including IFN-γ, when added to SEA-stimulated purified monocytes (FISCHER et al. 1990; GJÖRLOFF et al. 1991).

3 Binding Affinity Varies Among Different Species, Isotypes, and Allotypes

Although SAs are usually capable of activating the T cells of all mammalian species tested, there is considerable quantitative variation among different SEs in their affinity of interaction with the distinct MHC class II molecules, both when comparing the binding of different SEs to the same type of MHC class II molecules and when comparing the binding of the same SE to MHC class II molecules representing different species, isotypes, and allotypes (FISCHER et al. 1989; FRASER 1989; MOLLICK et al. 1989; HERRMANN et al. 1989; HERMAN et al. 1990; SCHOLL et al. 1990a; MARRACK and KAPPLER 1990). SEs generally bind with higher affinity to HLA-DR than to murine MHC class II antigens (HERMAN et al. 1990). In humans the highest affinity is observed with the HLA-DR isotype, whereas DQ and DP often show only a much weaker binding which is not always detectable in direct binding assays (FISCHER et al. 1989; FRASER 1989; UCHIYAMA et al. 1990). The strongest evidence for functional binding to the latter two comes from results using mouse fibroblast AC transfected with the MHC class II gene under study (MOLLICK et al. 1989; HERMAN et al. 1990; UCHIYAMA et al. 1990). Also, the alleles of DR vary greatly in their binding capacity for the same SE and for different SEs (HERMAN et al. 1990). Since HLA-DR molecules all share the same α-chain, these results imply that the DR β-chain has a dominating and determining role in SE binding and/or TCR interaction. Evidence has been provided, however, indicating that the α-chain is also of importance (LEE and WATTS 1990).

Analogous results have been recorded in mice demonstrating more efficient binding to I-E molecules, the murine counterpart to HLA-DR, than to I-A molecules, the homologue of HLA-DQ (UCHIYAMA et al. 1990). It has been suggested (HERMAN et al. 1990) that the greater efficiency of presentation on I-E (DR) might be related to the fact that this is the isotype serving as a ligand for SAs in the thymic selection, as exemplified by the Mls self SAs in the mouse (KAPPLER et al. 1987).

SEA has been shown to bind to purified murine I- E^d MHC class II molecules inserted in supported planar membranes (LEE and WATTS 1990). Specific binding of SEA to I-A^d was also observed, but the interaction was of significantly lower affinity. Binding of SEA to purified I-E^d was blocked by antibodies against both the α- and the β-chain of the I-E^d molecule, but not by antibodies specific for an unrelated MHC class II protein. Binding of SEA to I-A^d was blocked by an anti-Aβ^d- but not by an anti- Aα^d-specific antibody. Planar membranes containing only lipid and purified I-E^d molecules were sufficient for activation of a V$_\beta$1-expressing T hybrid by SEA. These data demonstrate that the purified MHC class II molecule is the only AC surface protein required for SEA binding and that MHC class II protein and intact SEA are both necessary and sufficient for T cell activation by the toxin, although other molecules of AC might enhance the induced T cell activation (KOTB et al. 1990; FLEISCHER et al. 1991; FISCHER et al. 1991). These data also confirm that SEA does not require processing for presentation to T cells. The weaker binding of SEA to I-A molecules was parallelled by a lower T cell response than that induced by SEA on I-E molecules. These results are consistent with reports that the SEA- and SEB-induced T cell response in mice cannot be totally blocked by either anti-I-E or anti-I-A alone but requires combined treatment with both antibodies (VROEGOP and BUXSER 1989). In the lipid membrane system the majority of purified I-E molecules were capable of binding SEA. At saturating conditions the number of SEA molecules bound to I-E was similar to the number of anti I-E antibodies bound, which indicates that SEA binds with an approximately 1:1 stoichiometry. In the case of streptococcal pyrogenic exotoxin type A (SPE A), activation of murine T cells also requires MHC class II molecules on AC (IMANISHI et al. 1990). In contrast to most other SEs, with this toxin I-A-transfected L cells functioned as well as I-E transfected and HLA class II transfected cells (IMANISHI et al. 1990).

Although TSST-1 has been shown to bind to all HLA-DR, -DQ, and -DP phenotypes tested (SCHOLL et al. 1990b), it shows an extremely variable binding to murine MHC class II molecules. It binds with high affinity to two of three I-A molecules (I-A^b and I- A^d) but only weakly to I-A^k and apparently not at all to two different I-E molecules (I- E^d and I-E^k). Similar results were reported by UCHIYAMA et al. (1989, 1990) showing that murine I-A and human DR and DQ molecules bind TSST-1 with similar affinities whereas I-E and DP molecules show no detectable binding in direct binding assays. The latter do function as AC, although at a lower level than the former molecules. This is in contrast to the functional binding of SEA to I-E transfectants of L cells but not to I-A transfectants (FLEISCHER et al. 1989). SCHOLL et al. (1990a) also studied transfected L cells expressing hybrid DR/I-E molecules and found that cells expressing DR$_\alpha$:I- E$^k_\beta$ but not I- E$^k_\alpha$:DR1$_\beta$ bound TSST-1 and supported T cell activation. This finding appears to indicate a major role for the α-chain of MHC class II in TSST-1 binding, but the difference in effect might also be conformational with the molecule exposing another critical TSST-1 binding site. Similar conclusions were drawn from the determination of the class II molecule region essential for high-affinity binding of TSST-1. This was done by direct binding experiments to different HLA-DR and -DP isotypes characterized by different affinities for the SE (KARP et al. 1990). By use of chimaeric α- and β-chains of DR and DP expressed at the surface of transfected murine fibroblasts, it was shown that the α-1 domain of DR is essential for high-affinity binding, whereas the α-chain of the DP had no such role. When the affinities of TSST-1 and SEB for MHC class II molecules were compared, the affinity of SEB was shown to be an order of magnitude lower (SCHOLL et al. 1989). It was further demonstrated by anti-HLA-DR antibody inhibition studies that the HLA class II molecule exhibits two distinct enterotoxin binding sites, one that is common for SEB and TSST-1 and another only used by TSST-1.

COLE et al. (1981) have shown that *Mycoplasma arthritidis*, a natural pathogen of rodents, produces a soluble T cell activator, MAM. This molecule has an absolute requirement for AC expressing functional I-E, whereas I-A in the absence of I-E does not suffice (COLE et al. 1982). I-E molecules extracted from B lymphoma cells and incorporated into liposomes can present MAM to T cells. Fibroblasts expressing intact I-E molecules after transfection with E-α and E-β genes could also present MAM to T cells (BEKOFF et al. 1987). Furthermore, by use of transfected fibroblasts expressing hybrid class II molecules and of mice expressing the transgenic E-α gene, it has been demonstrated that MAM is presented to T cells by I-E-α-containing molecules (COLE et al. 1990a, b).

Unlike other described SAs, the M protein of group A streptococci is a SA that was recently reported to stimulate exclusively human T cells but not T cells of other mammals (KOTB et al. 1990). It was also reported that the M protein can stimulate T cells in the absence of AC expressing HLA class II molecules, provided the costimulatory agents PMA, IL-1, and IL-6, interacting with immobilized or cross-linked protein M, are added. The same authors report analogous results with SEB. The M protein is of particular interest because of its presumed involvement in rheumatic fever and rheumatic heart disease. Similarly, FLEISCHER et al. (1989) have previously demonstrated that SEA induces T cells to proliferate in the presence of phorbol esters, though to a much lesser degree than in the presence of AC. CARLSSON et al. (1988) found no proliferation with highly purified T cells at low cell numbers (to further reduce the effect of the possibly remaining few contaminating AC) exposed to SEA and PMA but recorded IL-2 production. This appears to indicate that a partial T cell activation occurs in the absence of MHC class II expressing AC and that only a minor proliferative response is usually recorded even in the presence of PMA. Furthermore, even very few contaminating AC suffice for activation in the presence of PMA.

FLEISCHER et al. (1991) recently demonstrated that highly purified human resting T cells could be activated by streptococcal toxin A (ETA) and by SEB in the absence of AC, provided the T cells were exposed to immobilized toxin and anti-CD2 or anti-CD8 mAb on a solid phase (silica beads). These results are analogous to those obtained with certain anti-CD3 mAb which alone are not capable of stimulating T cell responses. These findings confirm that the toxins can indeed bind to the TCR in the absence of MHC class II molecules, but this is usually not sufficient for triggering of a T cell response without cross-linking with accessory molecules. Consistent with this view is the recent demonstration that the response of human naive CD45RA$^+$ CD4$^+$ T cells to SEA presented by HLA-DR transfected mouse fibroblasts was greatly enhanced by the simultaneous expression of ICAM-1 on the transfected fibroblasts (FISCHER et al. 1991).

4 Processing of SAs is not Required for T Cell Activation

That processing of SAs is not a requirement for T cell activation has been clearly demonstrated by the fact that AC treated with paraformaldehyde are often as effective in supporting T cell activation by SEA and TSST-1 as are untreated AC (CARLSSON et al. 1988). Although true for most SEs, this is not always the case; in particular paraformaldehyde- fixed L cell transfectants, irrespective of the MHC class II molecules expressed, have been reported to function only poorly as AC for murine and human T cells with, e.g., TSST-1, despite the maintained capacity to bind toxin (UCHIYAMA et al. 1990). This might indicate that in this case processing of the toxin heightens the AC activity of the cells, possibly by providing a more efficient interaction with the class II molecules or with the TCR. Alternatively, it might reflect the destruction of other accessory molecules that normally augment the interaction between the toxin and TCR. The recent demonstration that purified I-E molecules inserted in planar lipid bilayers were capable of binding SEA and of activating resting T cells and T cell hybridoma cells in the absence of AC (LEE and WATTS 1990) clearly establishes that there is no absolute requirement in this case for either toxin processing or any accessory molecule besides MHC class II itself. However, a few exceptional cases appear to exist in which processing is required. In the case of *Mycoplasma arthritidis* it has been reported that AC function is inhibited by the lysosomal inhibitors chloroquine and ammonium chloride or by the protease inhibitor leupeptin (BAUER et al. 1988). Also, *Pseudomonas aeruginosa* exotoxin A is claimed to require processing on the basis of a lack of AC function by paraformaldehyde- fixed cells when fixation is performed before toxin exposure but not when performed after (MISFELDT 1990).

5 Binding of SAs Occurs Outside the Antigen Groove of the MHC Class II Molecule

The question whether the same or different sites on the MHC class II molecules are used by different SAs has not yet been answered. SEA and SEB cross-compete for binding (FRASER 1989) and therefore probably bind to the same site on MHC or to sites in close proximity to each other, whereas SEB and TSST-1 do not (SCHOLL et al. 1989). The exact configuration of the toxin-class II complexes has not yet been clarified. By analogy with the established structure of MHC class I molecules (BJÖRKMAN et al. 1987), the structure of MHC class II molecules has been deduced. They are presumed to consist of two immunoglobulin-like domains located close to the cell lipid layer, supporting a part formed by the N-terminal regions of the two polypeptides of the protein and creating a groove in which peptides of foreign antigens are normally presented to the TCR. From the demonstration that association of SEB with mouse class II molecules does not inhibit the subsequent presentation of an authentic antigenic peptide derived from hen egg lysozyme to T cell clones (DELLABONA et al. 1990), it may be concluded that unprocessed bacterial toxins do not bind to MHC molecules by occupying this groove. This conclusion is also supported by the finding that TSST-1 binding did not prevent subsequent binding of a DR-restricted antigenic peptide (KARP et al. 1990).

T cells bearing closely related members of the same V-β family have been shown to respond differently to SE. This may be exemplified by the responsiveness to SEC2 of cells expressing the human V-β 13.2 element, whereas cells bearing the V-β 13.1 element are unresponsive (CHOI et al. 1990). The residues responsible for the 13.1/13.2 distinction were located to a region of TCR that is presumed to lie on the facet of the molecule that is outside of the conventional antigen binding groove. By directed mutagenesis experiments, the region of the TCR β-chain interacting with self SA Mls-1[a] was shown to reside outside the regions of the TCR that interact with conventional peptide antigens complexed with MHC (PULLEN et al. 1990).

6 Location of MHC Class II Binding Sites of SAs

Computer alignment of various enterotoxins has identified considerable and varying homologies, most prominently in the C-terminal rather than in the N-terminal part (MARRACK and KAPPLER 1990). It was reported that a 180 amino acid fragment of SEC1, obtained by deletion of the 59 N-terminal amino acids from the intact toxin molecule by digestion with trypsin, expressed the T mitogenic and pyrogenic properties of the molecule (BOHACH et al. 1989). This tends to indicate that for this toxin the N-terminal end of the molecule is not essential either for binding to MHC class II or for interaction with the TCR. Also, in the case of TSST-1, it has been shown that the MHC class II binding site(s) is located in the C-terminal part of the molecule (BLANCO et al. 1990; EDWIN and KASS 1989).

On the basis of experiments using synthetic small peptides and their respective antibodies, it has been concluded that SEA contains an MHC class II binding site in the N-terminal amino acids 1-27 (PONTZER et al. 1989). However, it was recently demonstrated that a C-terminal fragment of recombinant SEA, containing amino acids 107–233, binds to MHC class II, although it fails to activate human T cells (HEDLUND et al. 1991). The fragment bound to Raji cells expressing HLA class II but not to Raji cells lacking such expression. This fragment interfered with the subsequent binding and T cell activation by intact SEA. Binding of labeled fragment, cross-linking, and detergent solubilization of the cell membranes followed by electrophoresis demonstrated association of the fragment with MHC class II chains. Immunoprecipitation experiments showed that the fragment was associated with HLA-DR, -DQ, and -DP. Collectively these data seem to indicate that there are at least two HLA class II-binding sites in the SEA molecule, none of which involve any of the two cysteines of the molecule.

An attempt has recently been made to clarify the possible role of the disulfide loop and adjacent sequence of SEA and SEB (GROSSMAN et al. 1990). Breaking the sulfide loop by reduction and alkylation greatly reduced the T cell mitogenic activity of these SEs but did not destroy their capacity to bind to MHC class II molecules or their capacity to induce production of TNF-α from monocytes. Although the nature of the function of the loop was not clarified, these results may indicate a functional role for it. It is not known whether the importance of the loop is in providing a binding site for the TCR or rather in creating a conformation that results in a functional association between MHC binding and TCR binding sites located at some distance from each other. The latter possibility might be reconciled with the previously mentioned evidence for the involvement of the N-terminal end in T cell activation and the recent evidence of HLA class II binding of a C-terminal recombinant SEA fragment lacking T cell mitogenic activity.

Of great interest in relation to the affinity between the enterotoxins and the MHC class II molecules is the fact that there is a significant sequence homology between the human and murine invariant chains and certain SEs (MARRACK and KAPPLER 1990).

7 Importance of Molecules Other than MHC Class II for T Cell Activation

The existence of SA binding molecules distinctly different from MHC class II molecules is indicated by recent results demonstrating that SEB and SEC1, but not SEA and SED, were efficiently presented to cytotoxic lymphocytes (CTL) at picomolar concentrations by MHC class II-negative colon carcinoma cells (DOHLSTEN et al. 1991). The nature of the SE binding molecule expressed by these tumor cells has not yet been elucidated.

As already mentioned there are a number of molecules that function as accessory molecules in the binding and activation of T cells by SEs. Cross-linking of SE with CD2 and CD8, has been shown to replace AC (FLEISCHER et al. 1991). Anti-CD4 antibodies, but not anti-CD8, block T cell activation in mice (HEEG et al. 1991). Coexpression of ICAM-1 and HLA-DR on AC greatly enhances the SEA-induced T cell activation (FISCHER et al. 1991).

8 Possible Role of MHC Class II Molecules in SA-Induced T Cell Suppression

It has been reported that in vivo priming of mice with SEB abrogates the subsequent SEB in vitro response of V-$\beta 8^+$ CD4$^+$ (RELLAHAN et al. 1990) but not of V-$\beta 8^+$CD8$^+$ T cells (KAWABE and OCHI 1990). This might indicate that the CD4 molecule provides an accessory signal necessary for the generation of T cell anergy and would implicate a role of MHC class II-CD4 interaction in generation of this suppression. The mechanism is presumed to be either clonal deletion, analogous to that demonstrated in neonatally exposed mice (WHITE et al. 1989), or anergy induction. However, several reports suggest that SEB presented on MHC class II molecules stimulates T cells with suppressor activity resulting in inhibition of: (1) both primary and secondary plaque-forming cell (PFC) responses (DONNELLY and ROGERS 1982), (2) cytotoxic T cell activity (LIN et al. 1986), (3) secretion of antibody by a variety of plasmacytoma cell lines (LIN and ROGERS 1986), (4) first-set skin graft rejection responses (KAWAGUCHI- NAGATA et al. 1985), and (5) the delayed-type hypersensitivity (DTH) reaction to sheep erythrocytes (LIN et al. 1991). By use of I- J congenic mouse strains as a source of suppressor-effector and immune target populations, it has been established that the suppressor activity is restricted at the I-J gene locus (TAUB et al. 1990). Depletion analysis with anti-I-J mAb suggests that the suppressor-effector cells bear the I-J determinant on their surface. The suppression of DTH has been shown to be adoptively transferrable by $CD5^+$, $I-J^+$, $CD4^-$, $CD8^-$ T cells from SEB-treated mice. These results indicate that SEB-induced suppressor T cell populations are strikingly similar to previously described Ag-induced suppressor cells. At the present time the possible MHC class II involvement in the generation of these suppressive effects induced by certain SEs remains unclear.

9 Conclusions

T cells can interact directly with soluble SAs in the absence of AC, as revealed by a rapid increase in the cytosolic calcium ion concentration, but fail to become fully activated to IL-2 production and proliferation. MHC class II is the most essential molecule of AC. It allows optimal T cell activation since it alone is capable of binding the SA and presenting it unprocessed to the TCR in a form usually leading to a full activation of both $CD4^+$ and $CD8^+$ T cells. The role of the MHC class II molecule in T cell activation appears to be to enhance CD3 clustering by providing a multivalent SE and possibly to alter the SE conformation to increase the affinity to the V-β of TCR. SAs bind to MHC class II molecules on site(s) located outside of the peptide-presenting groove of these molecules. Other accessory molecules are of importance in augmenting T cell activation, probably by increasing the binding affinity and by cross-linking certain key molecules with the TCR. The interaction of SAs with certain AC leading to activation of cytokine release from these cells is less well understood but appears to be dependent on MHC class II expression on the AC and on T cell-derived molecules provided at the T cell surface or released from T cells. It has not yet been defined whether MHC class II molecules have a role in deciding whether the result of a T cell's intercourse with a SA will be a maintained expansion of the responding T cells, will be followed by programmed T cell death and selective elimination, or will result in the induction of anergy.

References

Bauer A, Rutenfranz I, Kirchner H (1988) Processing requirements for T cell activation by Mycoplasma arthritidis-derived mitogen. Eur J Immunol 18: 2109–2112

Bekoff MC, Cole BC, Grey HM (1987) Studies on the mechanism of stimulation of T cells by the Mycoplasma arthritidis derived mitogen. Role of class II I-E molecules. J Immunol 139: 3189–3194

Björkman PJ, Saper MA, Samraoui B, Bennett WS, Strominger JL, Wiley DC (1987) The foreign antigen binding site and T cell recognition regions of class I histocomapatibility antigens. Nature 329: 512–518

Blanco L, Choi EM, Connolly K, Thompson MR, Bonventre PF (1990) Mutants of staphylococcal toxic shock syndrome toxin 1; mitogenicity and recognition by a neutralizing monoclonal antibody. Infect Immun 58: 3020–3028

Bohach GA, Handley JP, Schlievert PM (1989) Biological and immunological properties of the carboxyl terminus of staphylococcal enterotoxin C1. Infect Immun 57: 23–28

Carlsson R, Fischer H, Sjögren HO (1988) Binding of staphylococcal enterotoxin A to accessory cells is a requirement for its ability to activate human T-cells. J Immunol 140: 2484–2488

Choi Y, Herman A, diGiusto D, Wade T, Marrack P, Kappler J (1990) Residues of the variable region of the T-cell receptor β-chain that interact with S. aureus toxin superantigens. Nature 346: 471–473

Cole BC, Daynes RA, Ward JR (1981) Stimulation of mouse lymphocytes by a mitogen derived from Mycoplasma arthritidis. I. Transformation is associated with an H-2-linked gene that maps to the I-E-I-C subregion. J Immunol 127: 1931–1936

Cole BC, Sullivan GJ, Daynes RA, Sayed IA, Ward JR (1982) Stimulation of mouse lymphocytes by a mitogen derived from Mycoplasma arthritidis. II. Cellular requirements for T cell transformation mediated by a soluble mycoplasma mitogen. J Immunol 128: 2013–2018

Cole BC, David CS, Lynch DH, Kartchner DR (1990a) The use of transfected fibroblasts and transgenic mice expressing Ealpha establishes that stimulation of $V_\beta8$ T cells by the Mycoplasma arthritidis mitogen requires Ealpha. J Immunol 144: 420–424

Cole BC, Kartchner DR, Wells DJ (1990b) Stimulation of mouse lymphocytes by a mitogen derived from Mycoplasma arthritidis (MAM). VIII. Selective activation of T cells expressing distinct V-T cell receptors from various strains of mice by the superantigen MAM. J Immunol 144: 425–431

Dellabona P, Peccoud J, Kappler J, Marrack P, Benoist C, Mathis D (1990) Superantigens interact with MHC class II molecules outside of the antigen groove. Cell 62: 1115–1121

Dohlsten M, Hedlund G, Segrén S, Lando PA, Herrmann T, Kelly AP, Kalland T (1991) Human MHC class II-colon carcinoma cells present staphylococcal superantigens to cytotoxic T lymphocytes: evidence for a novel enterotoxin receptor. Eur J Immunol 121: 131–135

Donnelly RP, Rogers TJ (1982) Immunosuppression induced by staphylococcal enterotoxin B. Cell Immunol 72: 166–173

Dyson PJ, Knight AM, Fairchild S, Simpson E, Tomonari K (1991) Genes encoding ligands for deletion of $V_\beta11$ T cells cosegregate with mammary tumor virus genomes. Nature 349: 531–532

Edwin C, Kass EH (1989) Identificiation of functional antigenic segments of toxic shock syndrome toxin 1 by differential immunoreactivity and by differential mitogenic responses of human peripheral blood mononuclear cells, using active toxin fragments. Infect Immun 57: 2230–2236

Fischer H, Dohlsten M, Lindvall M, Sjögren HO, Carlsson R (1989) Binding of staphylococcal enterotoxin A to HLA-DR on B cell lines. J Immunol 142: 3151–3157

Fischer H, Dohlsten M, Andersson U, Hedlund G, Ericsson PO, Hansson J, Sjögren HO (1990) Production of TNF-α and TNF-β by staphylococcal enterotoxin A activated human T cells. J Immunol 144: 4663–4669

Fischer H, Hedlund G, Gjörloff A, Hedman H, Lundgren E, Kalland T, Sjögren HO, Dohlsten M (1991) Stimulation of human naive and memory T helper cells with bacterial superantigen: Naive CD4+ 45RA+ T cells require a costimulatory signal mediated through the LFA-1/ICAM-1 pathway. (submitted)

Fleischer B, Schrezenmeier H (1988) T cell stimulation by staphylococcal enterotoxins. J Exp Med 167: 1697–1707

Fleischer B, Schrezenmeier H, Conradt P (1989) T cell stimulation by staphylococcal enterotoxin: role of class II molecules and T cell surface structure. Cell Immunol 119: 92–101

Fleischer B, Gerardy-Schahn R, Metzroth B, Carrel S, Gerlach D, Köhler W (1991) An evolutionary conserved mechanism of T cell activation by microbial toxins. Evidence for different affinities of T cell receptor-toxin interaction. J Immunol 146: 11–17

Frankel WN, Rudy C, Coffin JM, Huber BT (1991) Linkage of Mls genes to endogenous mammary tumor viruses of inbread mice. Nature 349: 526–528

Fraser JD (1989) High affinity binding of staphylococcal enterotoxins A and B to HLA-DR. Nature 339: 221–223

Gjörloff A, Fischer H, Hedlund G, Hansson J, Kenney JS, Allison AC, Sjögren HO, Dohlsten M (1991) Optimal induction of interleukin-1 in human monocytes by the superantigen staphylococcal enterotoxin A requires the participation of T helper cells. Cellular Immunol (in press).

Grossman D, Cook RG, Sparrow JT, Mollick JA, Rich RR (1990) Dissociation of the stimulatory activities of staphylococcal enterotoxins for T cells and monocytes. J Exp Med 172: 1831–1841

Hedlund G, Dohlsten M, Lando PA, Kalland T (1990) Staphylococcal enterotoxins direct and trigger CTL killing of autologous HLA-DR mononuclear leukocytes and freshly prepared leukemia cells. Cell Immunol 129: 426–434

Hedlund G, Dohlsten M, Buell G, Herrmann T, Lando PA, Segrén S, Schrimsher J, MacDonald HR, Sjögren HO, Kalland T (1991) A recombinant C-terminal fragment of SEA binds with high affinity to human MHC class II. (submitted)

Heeg K, Bendigs S, Bader P, Miethke T, Wagner H (1991) Reactivity of murine T-cell subsets against the superantigen staphylococcal enterotoxin B (SEB): identification of high frequent, high affinity, and MHC unrestricted cytotoxic T cell precursors in CD8$^+$ and CD4$^+$ T cells. (submitted)

Herman A, Croteau G, Sekaly RP, Kappler J, Marrack P (1990) HLA-DR alleles differ in their ability to present staphylococcal enterotoxins to T cells. J Exp Med 172: 709–717

Herrmann T, Accolla RS, MacDonald HR (1989) Different staphylococcal enterotoxins bind preferentially to distinct MHC class II isotypes. Eur J Immunol 19: 2171–2174

Herrmann T, Maryanski JL, Romero P, Fleischer B, MacDonald HR (1990) Activation of MHC class I-restricted CD8$^+$ CTL by microbial T cell mitogens. J Immunol 144: 1181–1186

Imanishi K, Igarashi H, Uchiyama T (1990) Activation of murine T cells by streptococcal pyrogenic exotoxin A. Requirement for MHC class II molecules on accessory cells and identification of V_β elements in T cell receptor of toxin-reactive T cells. J Immunol 144: 3170–3175

Janeway CA (1990) Self superantigens. Cell 63: 659–661

Jupin C, Anderson S, Damais C, Alouf JE, Parant M (1988) Toxic shock syndrome toxin 1 as an inducer of human tumor necrosis factors and gamma interferon. J Exp Med 167: 752–761

Kappler JW, Wade T, White J, Kushner E, Blackman M, Roehm BJ, Marrack P (1987) A T cell receptor V_β segment that imparts reactivity to a class II major histocompatibility complex product. Cell 49: 262–271

Karp DR, Teletski CL, Scholl P, Geha R, Long EO (1990) The alpha 1 domain of the HLA-DR molecule is essential for high-affinity binding of the toxic shock syndrome toxin-1. Nature 346: 474: 476

Kawabe Y, Ochi A (1990) Selective anergy of V_β^+, CD4$^+$ T cells in staphylococcus enterotoxin B—primed mice. J Exp Med 172: 1065–1070

Kawabe Y, Ochi A (1991) Programmed cell death and extrathymic reduction of $V_\beta 8^+$ CD4$^+$ T cells in mice tolerant to Staphylococcus aureus enterotoxin B. Science 349: 245–248

Kawaguchi-Nagata K, Okamura H, Shoji K, Kanagawa H, Semma M, Shinagawa K (1985) Immunomodulating activities of staphylococcal enterotoxins. I. Effects on in vivo antibody responses and contact sensitivity reaction. Microbiol Immunol 29: 183–193

Kotb M, Majumdar G, Tomai M, Beachey EH (1990) Accessory cell-independent stimulation of human T cells by streptococcal M protein superantigen. J Immunol 145: 1332–1336

Lee JM, Watts TH (1990) Binding of staphylococcal enterotoxin A to purified murine MHC class II molecules in supported lipid bilayers. J Immunol 145: 3360–3366

Lin YS, Rogers TJ (1986) Inhibition of antibody production from the plasmacytoma cell line MOPC-315 by staphylococcal enterotoxin B-induced T-suppressor cells. Cell Immunol 102: 299–306

Lin YS, Patel MR, Linna J, Rogers TJ (1986) Suppression of cytolytic T-cell activity by staphylococcal enterotoxin B-induced suppressor cells: role of interleukin 2. Cell Immunol 103: 147–159

Lin YS, Hu SC, Jan MS, Rogers TJ (1991) Inhibition of the delayed-type hypersensitivity response by staphylococcal enterotoxin B-induced suppressor T cells. Cell Immunol 132: 532–538

Marrack P, Kappler J (1990) The staphylococcal enterotoxins and their relatives. Science 248: 705–711

Marrack P, Kushnir E, Kappler J (1991) A maternally inherited superantigen encoded by a mammary tumor virus. Nature 349: 524–526

Misfeldt ML (1990) Microbial "superantigens". Infect Immun 58: 2409–2413

Mollick JA, Cook RG, Rich RR (1989) Class II MHC molecules are specific receptors for staphylococcal enterotoxin A. Science 244: 817–820

Mollick JA, Deemer KP, Rich RR (1990) MHC class II molecules transduce signals in monocytes in response to bound staphylococcal enterotoxin and toxic shock syndrome toxin. Clin Res 38: 305A

Peary DL, Adler WH, Smith RT (1970) The mitogenic effect of endotoxin and staphylococcal enterotoxin B on mouse spleen cells and human peripheral blood lymphocytes. J Immunol 105: 1453–1457

Pontzer CH, Russell JK, Johnson HM (1989) Localization of an immune functional site on staphylococcal enterotoxin A using the synthetic peptide approach. J Immunol 143: 280–284

Pullen AM, Wade T, Marrack P, Kappler JW (1990) Identification of the region of T cell receptor beta chain that interacts with the self-superantigens Mls-1a. Cell 61: 1365–1374

Rellahan BL, Jones LA, Kruisbeek AM, Fry AM, Matis LA (1990) In vivo induction of anergy in peripheral $V_\beta 8^+$ T cells by staphylococcal enterotoxin B J Exp Med 172: 1091–1100

Scholl PR, Diez A, Geha RS (1989) Staphylococcal enterotoxin B and toxic shock syndrome toxin-1 bind to distinct sites on HLA-DR and HLA-DQ molecules. J Immunol 143: 2583–2588

School PR, Diez A, Karr R, Seakaly RP, Trowsdale J, Geha RS (1990a) Effect of isotypes and allelic polymorphism on the binding of staphylococcal enterotoxins to MHC class II molecules. J. Immunol 144: 226–230

Scholl PR, Sekaly RP, Diez A, Glimcher LH, Geha RS (1990b) Binding of toxic shock syndrome toxin-1 to murine major histocompatibility complex class II molecules. Eur J Immunol 20: 1911–1916

Taub DD, Lin YS, Rogers TJ (1990) Characterization and genetic restriction of suppressor-effector cells induced by staphylococcal enterotoxin B J Immunol 144: 456–462

Uchiyama T, Imanishi K, Saito S, Araake M, Yan XJ, Fujikawa H, Igarashi H, Kato H, Obata F, Kashiwagi N, Inoko H (1989a) Activation of human T cells by toxic shock syndrome toxin-1: the toxin-binding structures expressed on human lymphoid cells acting as accessory cells are HLA class II molecules. Eur J Immunol 19: 1803–1809

Uchiyama T, Tadakuma T, Imanishi K, Araake M, Saito S, Yan XJ, Fujikawa H, Igarashi H, Yamaura N (1989b) Activation of murine T cells by toxic shock syndrome toxin-1. J Immunol 143: 3175–3182

Uchiyama T, Saito S, Inoko H, Yan XJ, Imanishi K, Araake M, Igarashi H (1990) Relative activities of distinct isotypes of murine and human major histocompatibility complex class II molecules in binding toxic shock syndrome toxin 1 and determination of CD antigens expressed on T cells generated upon stimulation by the toxin. Infect Immun 58: 3877–3882

Vroegop SM, Buxser SE (1989) Cell surface molecules involved in early events in T-cell mitogenic stimulation by staphylococcal enterotoxin . Infect Immun 57: 1816–1824

White J, Herman A, Pullen AM, Kubo R, Kappler JW, Marrack P (1989) The V_β-specific superantigen staphylococcal enterotoxin B: stimulation of mature T cells and clonal deletion in neonatal mice. Cell 56: 27–35

Woodland DL, Happ MP, Gollob KJ, Palmer E (1991) An endogenous retrovirus mediating deletion of alpha/beta T cells. Nature 349: 529–530

The Human T Cell Response to Mitogenic Microbial Exotoxins

B. FLEISCHER

1 Introduction

Nearly every infectious pathogen has to cope with the host's adaptive immune response. Common evasion mechanisms in this complex interaction are antigenic variations, the escape to immunologically privileged sites, or the use of immunosuppressive mechanisms. Many bacteria and other microorganisms elaborate soluble factors or toxins that act suppressively on cells of the immune system, such as pore-forming molecules or proteins that interfere with the function of G proteins. Gram-positive cocci and a mycoplasma have developed an extremely potent mechanism of T cell stimulation by closely mimicking recognition of specific antigen. From the functional similarity to antigen recognition and the multiclonal activation of T cells, the designation "superantigen" has been suggested for these molecules (WHITE et al. 1989). This review will focus on the action of the microbial toxins on human T cells.

2 Mitogenic Toxins

Table 1 lists all proteins that have until today reported to be superantigens. Major producers are gram-positive cocci but also two distant microorganisms produce T cell stimulating proteins that could fall into the superantigen category. The

Pathophysiology Section, First Department of Medicine, University of Mainz, 6500 Mainz, FRG

Table 1. Microbial products implicated as superantigens

Protein Name	Abbreviation	Producing microorganism	M_r	Stimulatory Concentrations (ng/ml)	Reported preference for human V_β
Enterotoxin A	SEA	S. aureus	27 800	0.1–1	3, 12, 14, 15, 17, 20
B	SEB		28 300	1–10	
C_1	SEC_1		26 000	1–10	
C_2	SEC_2		26 000	1–10	12, 17, 13.1
C_3	SEC_3		28 900	1–10	
D	SED		27 300	0.1–1	
E	SEE		29 600	0.1–1	
Toxic shock syndrome toxin-1	TSST-1		22 000	1–10	8
Exfoliative toxin A	ExFTA		26 950	ND	2
B	ExFTB		27 300	ND	2
Erythrogenic toxin A	ETA	S. pyogenes	29 200	0.1–1	ND
B	ETB		27 000	1000	8
C	ETC		24 300	0.01–1	8
M protein	pepM		33 000	1000	8
Exotoxin A		P. aeruginosa	66 000	10–100	ND
Soluble mitogen	MAM	M. arthritidis	~15 000	~1–10	ND

prototypes are the genetically related staphylococcal enterotoxins (SE) that can be distinguished by neutralizing antisera. Most of the SE do not cross-react with other members of the SE family. The erythrogenic toxins A and C of *S. pyogenes* also belong to this family.

For an unequivocal demonstration that a given microbial toxin is a superantigen which uses the MHC class II-dependent mechanism described below, it has to be demonstrated that the isolated protein shares the typical characteristics of the SE:

1. Activity in nanomolar concentrations
2. Specific binding to MHC class II molecules
3. Clonal heterogeneity of the T cell response

It has recently been demonstrated that the staphylococcal protein A is not a T cell mitogen but that its T cell stimulatory activity is due to minute contaminations by SE. Antibodies to SEA and SEB block specifically the T cell response to protein A, and protein A produced in *E. coli* is not mitogenic (SCHREZENMEIER and FLEISCHER 1987).

Due to the extreme potency of the SE and the streptococcal ET, the possibility must always be considered that the superantigenic nature of novel staphylococcal or streptococcal proteins could be due to contaminating SE or ET. It should be noted in this context that the epidermolytic exfoliative toxins (ExFT) have no homologies to the SE family and that MHC class II binding was not detected with the ExFT A (HERRMANN et al. 1989). We have not been able to detect any mitogenicity with recombinant ExFTA (unpublished observations). In addition, the features of the streptococcal M protein suspiciously resemble that of the streptococcal ET (BRAUN et al. 1991). Such contaminations can be excluded in the case of the *Mycoplasma arthritidis* mitogen MAM (ATKIN et al. 1986) and the *Pseudomonas aeruginosa* exotoxin A. MAM shares all the characteristics of the SE (MATTHES et al. 1988; COLE et al. 1990) and is definitely a superantigen. *Pseudomonas aeruginosa* exotoxin A, an ADP-ribosylating toxin that has T lymphocyte stimulating activity (ZEHAVI-WILLNER 1988; MISFELDT 1990), has not been studied in sufficient detail to establish its superantigenic character. A possible acquisition of such toxins by microorganisms other than gram-positive cocci can be envisaged because the toxins are encoded by mobile genetic elements (see the chapter by LEE and SCHLIEVERT, this volume).

3 Molecular Mechanism of T Cell Stimulation by SE

Stimulation of T cells with SE is absolutely dependent on the presence of monocytes as "accessory" cells (ACs). Monocytes as ACs can be replaced by cells of many different types but only if they express MHC class II molecules (FLEISCHER and SCHREZENMEIER 1988; JANEWAY et al. 1989). In the presence of MHC class II-negative cells, T cells are unresponsive to SE. That indeed expression of MHC class II molecules is the critical property of ACs can be shown by transfection: a nonstimulating cell is rendered stimulatory for SE-induced T cell activation if transfected with a cloned MHC class II gene (FLEISCHER et al. 1989). This requirement for MHC class II molecules is apparently different from the MHC-restricted antigen recognition, since any class II-positive ACs can stimulate most T cell clones in the presence of most SE. Even murine T cells can respond to human class II-positive ACs and vice versa.

Another indication that the T cell response to SE was unrelated to MHC-restricted antigen recognition was the finding that CD8$^+$ T cells that usually respond to antigen in association with class I molecules also require MHC class II molecules for their response to SE (FLEISCHER and SCHREZENMEIER 1988). Similarly, $\gamma\delta$TCR$^+$ T cells were found that could also respond to SEA in a class II-dependent manner. It is noteworthy that SE are extremely potent inducers of cytotoxicity against MHC class II-positive target cells.

For stimulation of T cells by SE, a binding of the intact toxin molecule to MHC class II molecules is required and sufficient. There is no need for processing of the toxin because fixed AC stimulate as well as unfixed cells. The toxins bind selectively to MHC class II molecules with affinities of 10^{-6}–10^{-7} M (FISCHER et al. 1989; FRAZER 1989; MOLLIK et al. 1989), but outside the antigen-binding groove (DELLABONNA et al. 1990). Some toxins have different affinities for different isotypes and allotypes of class II molecules, indicating that polymorphic parts of both α and β chains of class II molecules influence binding to the toxins (HERMAN et al. 1990; SCHOLL 1990). Generally, SE bind with higher affinity to human than to murine class II molecules (HERMAN et al. 1990).

In contrast to conventional mitogens, e.g., lectins, a given toxin does not stimulate every T cell. For example, at the clonal level, some T cells do not respond to SEA but do respond to SEB. Furthermore, different T cell clones appear to react with different toxins with variable affinities (FLEISCHER et al. 1991). In spite of the requirement for class II molecules in T cell stimulation, there is evidence that SE interact with the T cell receptor (TCR) directly, i.e., in the absence of class II molecules. This interaction is of low activity and is insufficient to generate a full response of the T cell. However, second messenger production, a rise in cytosolic Ca^{2+} and other evidence for direct action on the T cell can be detected (CHATILA et al. 1988; FLEISCHER et al. 1989, 1991).

Based on our own results, we proposed, in 1987 (FLEISCHER and SCHREZENMEIER 1987, 1988; MATTHES et al. 1988), that SE are functionally bivalent molecules binding to MHC class II molecules and to variable parts of TCR molecules present on $\alpha\beta$ and $\gamma\delta$ T cells. Similar but in details differing models have been developed by other groups (MARRACK and KAPPLER 1990; JANEWAY et al. 1989).

Such a model would predict that the interaction sites for TCR and class II molecules should be distinguishable. A recent report supports this notion. After reduction and alkylation of the disulfide loop, SEA and SEB still interact with class II molecules but fail to stimulate T cells (GROSSMAN et al. 1990). Thus, class II and TCR binding activities can be dissociated.

4 Basis of Clonal Heterogeneity

Stimulation of murine or human T cells with a given toxin in vitro leads to selective expansion of T cells carrying certain V_β (WHITE et al. 1989; JANEWAY et al. 1989). In cultures of murine spleen cells stimulation with, e.g., SEB leads to enrichment of $V_\beta 8^+$ T cells. Injection of SEB into neonatal mice leads to intrathymic deletion of $V_\beta 8$-bearing thymocytes (WHITE et al. 1989). A similar preference was reported by RUST et al. (1990) for the response of $\gamma\delta^+$ T cells; here, a response to SEA was found only with T cell clones bearing $V_\gamma 9$. That indeed the response to a given toxin can be critically dependent on the V_β was shown by CHOI et al. (1990). The introduction of eight amino acids of the human $V_\beta 13.2$ into the human $V_\beta 13.1$ was sufficient to confer SEC_2 reactivity to a T cell hybridoma. These amino acids are located at a site of V_β probably not involved in peptide antigen recognition.

However, a given V_β does not confer *specificity* for a given toxin. Stimulation of human T cells with, e.g., the ETs of *S. pyogenes* leads to a preferential expansion of $V_\beta 8^+$ T cells and depletion of $V_\beta 5^+$ T cells (FLEISCHER et al. 1991). If, however, cloned T cells carrying $V_\beta 5$ or $V_\beta 8$ were investigated it was found that $V_\beta 5^+$ T cells could respond to the ETs, although these T cells were depleted from bulk cultures after stimulation with these toxins. A likely explanation is that different TCRs bind to these toxins with different affinities and that T cells with the highest affinity for a given toxin are preferentially expanded. Apparently, the toxins are not specific for but rather show a preferential reactivity with certain TCRs. This notion is supported by the finding that more than 50% of human T cells react with a given toxin (FLEISCHER et al. 1991). An exception is the mitogen derived from *M. arthritidis* that only stimulates less than 5% of human T cells (MATTHES et al. 1988; FLEISCHER et al. 1991).

The structural requirements for the toxins are still unclear. Apparently, the interactions with class II molecules or TCRs are not mediated by linear parts of the molecule, because even large fragments fail to stimulate (FRAZER 1989). Deletion mutants of SEB show loss of mitogenic activity already after deletion of a few N-terminal or C-terminal amino acids far from the homologous parts of the different toxins (METZROTH et al. 1991). This indicates that a proper three-dimensional structure is required for activity.

Apparently, minor changes in the amino acid sequence of a toxin change its reactivity with the T cell. SEA and SEE have the highest homology (nearly 90%) among all toxins (COUCH et al. 1988) but can easily be distinguished by $V_\beta 8$ T cells (FLEISCHER et al. 1991). Nonetheless, the overall mechanism of T cell activation is very similar even with very unrelated molecules such as toxic shock syndrome toxin-1 (TSST-1) and the SE.

TSST-1 has only a few regions of homology with the SE, confined to spots of one or two amino acids. Such amino acids are possible markers for functionally important regions of the molecules. It is noteworthy that a mutation in amino acid 144, which is conserved between the SE, ET, and TSST-1, leads to both a loss of function and of immune reactivity with a monoclonal antibody (BLANCO et al.

1990). Thus, SE and related toxins act as intact three-dimensionally folded proteins cross-linking with distinct regions of the toxin molecule, TCR and MHC class II.

This cross-linking of the TCR, however, is not sufficient for T cell activation per se. Additional prerequisites are adhesions via CD2 and lymphocyte-function-associated antigen-1 (LFA-1) between T cells and ACs. Interestingly, because antibodies to CD2 or LFA-1 must be added together to inhibit completely (MITTRÜCKER et al. 1991). On CD8$^+$ T cells the response is not inhibitable by anti-CD8 antibodies even at higher concentrations. In contrast, some but not all CD4$^+$ T cell clones can be inhibited to some extent by anti-CD4 (FLEISCHER et al. 1989). Apparently, the CD4 and CD8 molecules are not essential coreceptors in the response to SE.

Furthermore, there is evidence for a clone-specific interaction between T cell and stimulator cell in the activation by the toxins. A given combination of T cell, AC, and toxin can be nonstimulatory although the same T cell can respond to the same toxin on another AC and although the same AC can present the same toxin to another T cell (FLEISCHER and MITTRÜCKER 1991). This indicates that in the complex formed between TCR, toxin, and class II molecule an interaction between TCRs and class II molecules takes place.

5 Enterotoxic Activity of SE

The SE are known and named for their ability to induce a gastrointestinal illness within 2–4 h after oral uptake of a few micrograms of toxin. The symptoms of the gastrointestinal intoxication are apparently caused by histamine and leukotrienes released from mast cells in the mucosa (SCHEUBER et al. 1985). Intradermal injection of SEB causes a skin reaction of anaphylactic type within a few minutes. This dermal reaction is caused by the same mediators and mechanisms as the enteric reaction. Both reactions are inducible only in primates, whereas mitogenicity is found in a wider range of species (SCHEUBER et al. 1985). The stimulation of mast cells in these reactions is indirect, probably mediated by substance P. SE probably act on intramucosal sensory ganglial cells that release neuropeptides in response to SE, because either antibodies to substance P or capsaicin pretreatment block the response to SEB (ALBER et al. 1989).

It thus appears that the enteropathogenic activity of SE is not caused by an action on T cells. This notion is supported by the finding that SEB carboxylmethylated on histidine residues completely loses its emetic activity but is still as mitogenic as the unmodified toxins (ALBER et al. 1990). Furthermore, a monoclonal anti-idiotypic antibody against the combining site of a neutralizing anti-SEB antibody blocks the enteric and skin response to a more than 10 000-fold molar excess of SEB in monkeys (RECK et al. 1988). This indicates a high-affinity binding to the putative SEB receptor in the skin and the gastric mucosa.

The anti-idiotype has no agonistic activity in the skin or in the gut. This antibody binds to T cells with very low affinity and is mitogenic for T cells similar to an anti-TCR antibody (ALBER et al. 1990). Taken together this indicates that SEB may recognize a related but not identical receptor structure on T cells and, possibly, neuronal cells in primates.

6 Mechanisms of Pathogenicity

Given the extremely low concentration (pg/ml) required for T cell stimulation and the large amounts of toxin secreted by these bacteria into the culture medium in vitro, it is clear that a small focus of bacterial infection can be sufficient to flood the immune system with toxin.

Introduction of a mitogenic toxin into the body may have a number of consequences. Polyclonal T cell stimulation can lead to immunosuppression because stimulation of many T cells will impede a coordinate immune response that requires specific cell-cell interactions. Most importantly, a toxin can induce anergy in those T cells responding to it (RELLAHAN et al. 1990; KAWABE and OCHI 1990). After injection of SEB into mice, $V_{\beta}8^+$ T cells are still present in the circulation but no longer respond to SEB or to anti-TCR antibodies. The response of other non-SEB-reactive T cells is not affected. In addition, activated $CD8^+$ T cells could destroy antigen presenting cells (APC) or B cells that have bound toxin molecules via their MHC class II antigens.

The shock-like symptoms induced by many of these toxins are caused by massive release of lymphokines and monokines. Similar symptoms are observed after the first injection of stimulating anti-CD3 antibodies in patients requiring immunosuppressive therapy. The mediator release from mast cells is likely to contribute to these conditions. Finally, these toxins could induce immunopathological phenomena. Autoreactive T cells could be nonspecifically activated or irrelevant T cells could be focused on autoreactive B cells and induce autoantibody production. It is noteworthy in this context that for the streptococcal toxins an association with rheumatic fever has been suggested (YU and FERRETTI 1989).

7 Concluding Remarks

The toxins described in this review constitute the most efficient T cell stimulators known. Conceivably, immunosuppression, destruction of APC, and T cell anergy will be of major advantage to the infecting microorganisms. The finding that the toxins derived from *S. aureus* and *S. pyogenes* (bacteria found only in humans) stimulate human T cells more efficiently than murine T cells, whereas the opposite is true for the mitogen derived from *M. arthritidis* (a natural pathogen for rodents) suggests that these molecules have been adapted in evolution to the MHC and TCR molecules of the natural host. The finding that: (a) only certain TCRs are addressed by a given toxin via variable parts and (b) not all T cells are addressed via a constant part of.the TCR reduces the in vivo efficacy of the toxins. However, this strategy prevents the induction of cross-reacting neutraliz-ing antibodies. Thus, the molecules of the enterotoxin family show a maximum of biological efficacy combined with a minimum of immunological cross-reactivity. This feature is the reason for the conservation of their polymorphism during evolution.

Note. Since completion of this manuscript several groups reported that the endogenous superantigens present in certain strains of mice are encoded by endogenous retroviruses (JANEWAY, C.A., *Nature* 349, 459, 1991). Thus these endogenous T cell stimulating determinants are derived from infectious pathogens similar to the exogenous superantigens of *S. aureus*, *S. pyogenes*, and *M. arthritidis*. Apparently, Mls and other retroviral superantigens are not conserved by certain murine strains to convey protection against autoimmune diseases or microbial toxins. Instead all these molecules are part of a strategy of infectious agents used to suppress the immune response by clonal deletion or anergy.

References

Alber G, Scheuber PH, Reck B, Sailer-Kramer B, Hartmann A, Hammer DK (1989) Role of substance P in immediate-type skin reactions induced by staphylococcal enterotoxin B in unsensitized monkeys. J Allergy Clin Immunol 84: 880–885

Alber G, Hammer DK, Fleischer B (1990) Relationship between enterotoxic and T lymphocyte stimulating activity of staphylococcal enterotoxin B. J Immunol 144: 4501–4506

Atkin CL, Cole BC, Sullivan GJ, Washburn LR, Wiley BB (1986) Stimulation of mouse lymphocytes by a mitogen derived from *M. arthritidis*. V. A small basic protein from culture supernatant is a potent T cell mitogen. J Immunol 137: 1581–1589

Bergdoll MS (1983) Enterotoxins. In: Easmon SCF, Adlams C (eds) Staphylococci and staphylococcal infections. Academic, New York, pp 559–598

Blanco L, Choi EM, Connolly K, Thompson MR, Bonventre PF (1990) Mutants of staphylococcal toxic shock syndrome toxin-1: mitogenicity and recognition by a neutralizing monoclonal antibody. Infect Immun 58: 3020–3028

Braun MA, Gerlach D, Ozegowski JH, Carre S, Köhler W, Fleischer B (1991) Preferential stimulation of $V_{\beta}8^+$ human T cells by the streptococcal "superantigens" erythrogenic toxins A and C (scarlet fever toxins). (submitted)

Chatila T, Wood N, Parsonnet J, Geha RS (1988) Toxic shock syndrome toxin-1 induces inositol phospholipid turnover, protein kinase C translocation and calcium mobilization in human T cells. J Immunol 140: 1250–1255

Choi Y, Herman A, DiGiusto D, Wade T, Marrack P, Kappler J (1990) Residues of the variable region of the T cell receptor β-chain that interact with *S. aureus* toxin superantigens. Nature 346: 471–473

Cole BC, Kartchener DC, Wells DJ (1990) Stimulation of mouse T lymphocytes by a mitogen derived from *Mycoplasma arthritidis*. VIII. Selective activation of T cells expressing distinct V_β T cell receptors from various strains of mice by the "superantigen" MAM. J Immunol 144: 425–429

Couch JL, Soltis MT, Betley MJ (1988) Cloning and nucleotide sequence of the type E staphylococcal enterotoxin gene. J Bacteriol 170: 2954–2960

Dellabonna P, Peccoud J, Kappler J, Marrack P, Benoist C, Mathis D (1990) Superantigens interact with MHC molecules outside the binding groove. Cell 62: 1115–1121

Fischer H, Dohlsten M, Lindvall M, Sjögren O, Carlsson R (1989) Binding of staphylococcal enterotoxin A to HLA-DR on B cell lines. J Immunol 142: 3151–3157

Fleischer B, Mittrücker HW (1991) Evidence for T cell receptor-HLA class II molecule interaction in the response to superantigenic bacterial toxins. Eur J Immunol 21: 1331–1333

Fleischer B, Schrezenmeier H (1987) Staphylococcal enterotoxins: MHC class II- dependent probes for the T cell antigen receptor. Immunobiology 175: 328–329

Fleischer B, Schrezenmeier H (1988) Stimulation by staphylococcal enterotoxins. Clonally variable response and requirement for MHC class II molecules on accessory or target cells. J Exp Med 167: 1697–1708

Fleischer B, Schrezenmeier H, Conradt P (1989) T cell stimulation by staphylococcal enterotoxins. Role of class II molecules and T cell surface structures. Cell Immunol 119: 92–101

Fleischer B, Gerardy-Schahn R, Metzroth B, Carrel S, Gerlach D, Köhler W (1991) A conserved mechanism of T cell stimulation by microbial toxins. Evidence for different affinities of T cell receptor-toxin interaction. J Immunol 146: 11–17

Frazer JD (1989) High affinity binding of staphylococcal enterotoxins A and B to HLA-DR. Nature 339: 221–223

Grossman D, Cook RD, Sparrow JT, Mollick JA Rich RR (1990) Dissociation of the stimulatory activities of staphylococcal enterotoxins for T cells and monocytes. J Exp Med 172: 1831–1841

Herman A, Croteau G, Sekaly RP, Kappler J, Marrack P (1990) HLA-DR alleles differ in their ability to present staphylococcal enterotoxins to T cells. J Exp Med 172: 709–717

Herrmann T, Acolla RS, MacDonald HR (1989) Different staphylococcal enterotoxins bind preferentially to distinct MHC class II isotypes. Eur J Immunol 19: 2171–2174

Janeway CA, Yagi J, Conrad PJ, Katz ME, Jones B, Vroegop S, Buxser S (1989) T cell responses to Mls and to bacterial proteins that mimic its behaviour. Immunol Rev 107: 61–68

Kappler J, Kotzin B, Herron L, Gelfand E, Bigler RD, Boylston A, Carrel S, Posneit DN, Choi Y, Marrack P (1989) V_β-specific stimulation of human T cells by staphylococcal toxins. Science 244: 811–814

Kawabe Y, Ochi A (1990) Selective anergy of V_β^+ CD4$^+$ T cells in staphylococcus enterotoxin B-primed mice. J Exp Med 172: 1065–1070

Marrack P, Kappler J (1990) The staphylococcal enterotoxins and their relatives. Science 248: 705–711

Matthes M, Schrezenmeier H, Homfeld J, Fleischer S, Malissen B, Kirchner H, Fleischer B (1988) Clonal analysis of human T cell activation by the *Mycoplasma arthritidis* mitogen. Eur J Immunol 18: 1733–1737

Metzroth B, Linnig M, Fleischer B (1991) Effect of deletions on function and antigenicity of staphylococcal enterotoxin B. (submitted)

Misfeldt ML (1990) Microbial "superantigens". Infect Immun 58: 2409–2413

Mittrücker H-W, Fleischer B (1991) Stimulator cell-dependent requirement for CD2 or LFA-1 mediated adhesions in the T cell response to superantigenic toxins. (submitted)

Mollik JA, Cook GR, Rich RG (1989) Class II MHC molecules are specific receptors for staphylococcal enterotoxin A. Science 244: 817

Reck B, Scheuber PH, Londong D, Sailer-Kramer B, Bartsch K, Hammer DK (1988) Protection against the staphylococcal enterotoxin-induced intestinal disorder in the monkey by anti-idiopathic antibodies. Proc Natl Acad Sci USA 85: 3170–3174

Rellahan BL, Jones LA, Kruisbeck AM, Fry AM, Mathis LA (1990) In vivo induction of anergy in peripheral $V_\beta 8^+$ T cells by staphylococcal enterotoxin B. J Exp Med 172: 1091–1100

Rust CJ, Verreck F, Vietor H, Koning F (1990) Specific recognition of staphylococcal enterotoxin A by human T cells bearing receptors with the $V_\gamma 9$ region. Nature 346: 572–574

Scheuber PH, Golecki JR, Kickhöfen B, Scheel D, Beck G, Hammer DK (1985) Skin reactivity of unsensitized monkeys upon challenge with staphylococcal enterotoxin B: a new approach for investigating the site of toxin action. Infect Immun 50: 869–876

Scholl PR, Sekaly RP, Diez A, Glimcher LM, Geha RS (1990) Binding of toxic shock syndrome toxin 1 to murine MHC class II molecules. Eur J Immunol 20: 1911–1916

Schrezenmeier H, Fleischer B (1987) Mitogenic activity of staphylococcal protein A is due to contaminating staphylococcal enterotoxins. J Immunol Methods 105: 133–137

Tomai M, Kotb M, Majumdjar G, Beachey EH (1990) Superantigenicity of streptococcal M protein. J Exp Med 172: 359–362

White J, Herman A, Pullen AM, Kubo R, Kappler JW, Marrack P (1989) The V_β-specific superantigen staphylococcal enterotoxin B: stimulation of mature T cells and clonal deletion in neonatal mice. Cell 56: 27–35

Yu C, Ferretti J (1989) Molecular epidemiologic analysis of the type A streptococcal exotoxin in clinical *S. pyogenes* strains. Infect Immun 57: 3715–3719

Zehavi-Willner (1988) Induction of murine cytolytic T lymphocytes by *Pseudomonas aeruginosa* exotoxin A. Infect Immunol 56: 213–218

Toxic Shock Syndrome Toxin-1, Toxic Shock, and the Immune System

T. Chatila, P. Scholl, F. Spertini, N. Ramesh, N. Trede, R. Fuleihan, and R. S. Geha

1 Introduction

Toxic shock syndrome (TSS) is a severe multisystem disorder characterized by high fever, hypotension, generalized erythroderma, desquamation of the skin, and dysfunction of multiple organ systems (Chesney 1989; Davis et al. 1980; Todd et al. 1978). TSS is consistently associated with infection by toxigenic strains of *Staphylococcus aureus*, most commonly in the setting of tampon use during menses or following surgery or trauma. Exotoxins secreted by staphylococcal isolates from patients with TSS, most notably toxic shock syndrome toxin-1 (TSST-1), but also the structurally related staphylococcal enterotoxins, play a key role in the pathophysiology of this disease. It has been recently appreciated that the toxicity of TSST-1 stems from its ability to initiate uncontrolled activation of large numbers of immune cells by virtue of its capacity to bind MHC class II (Ia) molecules (Scholl et al. 1989a; Uchiyama et al. 1989a). Once bound to Ia molecules, TSST-1 can transmit activation signals to Ia$^+$ immune cells including

Division of Immunology, The Children's Hospital and the Department of Pediatrics, Harvard Medical School, Boston, MA 02115, USA monocytes, B lymphocytes, activated T lymphocytes, and activated natural killer cells. At the same time, Ia-bound TSST-1 acts as a superantigen that interacts with and activates human T lymphocytes whose T cell receptor β chains bear a particular variable (V) gene sequence, $V_{\beta}2$ (CHOI et al. 1989). In this review, we will focus on the characteristics of the interaction between TSST-1 and Ia molecules and on the functional consequences of superantigen formation, including V_{β}-restricted activation of T lymphocytes and superantigen-mediated cognate T/B cell interaction. We will also examine evidence for the induction by TSST-1 of transmembrane signals via Ia molecules that regulate intercellular adhesion interactions mediated by lymphocyte function-associated molecule 1 (LFA-1; CD11a/CD18), T and B lymphocyte activation, and monokine gene transcription. Finally, we will discuss the relevance of the interaction of TSST-1 with Ia molecules to the pathophysiology of TSS.

2 Role of TSST-1 and Related Exotoxins in TSS

Unlike randomly tested staphylococcal isolates, the overwhelming majority of staphylococcal isolates from patients with TSS are toxigenic (BERGDOLL et al. 1981; BONVENTRE et al. 1989; CRASS and BERGDOLL 1986; SCHLIEVERT et al. 1981). Almost all staphylococcal isolates from menstruation-associated toxic shock syndrome patients and half of the isolates from nonmenstrual toxic shock syndrome patients express TSST-1 alone or, more commonly, in combination with one or more of the staphylococcal enterotoxins (CRASS and BERGDOLL 1986). The majority of TSST-1 negative isolates express one or more of the staphy-lococcal enterotoxins, particularly staphylococcal enterotoxin B (SEB) (CRASS and BERGDOLL 1986; PARSONNET et al. 1986; SCHLIEVERT 1986). The critical role played by TSST-1 in the genesis of TSS has been established by studies demonstrating that TSST-1-positive strains of *Staphylococcus aureus* produce a TSS-like illness in rabbits, while isogenic TSST-1- negative strains fail to do so (DE AZAVEDO et al. 1985; RASHEED et al. 1985). Passive immunization with a neutraliz-ing anti-TSST-1 monoclonal antibody protects rabbits from otherwise lethal infection with TSST-1 producing strains of staphylococci (BEST et al. 1988). Further evidence incriminating TSST-1 in the pathogenesis of TSS came from the demonstration that constant infusion of purified TSST-1 in rabbits also produces a TSS-like illness (PARSONNET et al. 1987) and that rabbits can be protected against this illness by passive immunization with the same neutralizing anti-TSST-1 monoclonal antibody (BONVENTRE et al. 1988). Interestingly, infusion of staphylococcal entertoxins induces a TSS-like illness in rabbits indistinguishable from that following TSST-1 infusion (PARSONNET et al. 1987). This supported a role for staphylococcal enterotoxins in the pathogenesis of TSS, especially in cases associated with enterotoxin-producing but TSST-1-nonproducing strains of staphylococci.

The susceptibility to TSS seems to correlate with poor antibody response to TSST-1 and to enterotoxins (CRASS and BERGDOLL 1986). Thus, while the majority of healthy individuals have protective titers of antibodies against TSST-1, more than 80% of patients with TSS display no detectable levels of anti-TSST-1 antibodies when examined during the acute phase of the disease. Furthermore, most TSS patients fail to develop protective titers of anti-TSST-1 antibodies following convalescence. A similar trend was observed when examining titers of anti-enterotoxin antibodies. This suggested that most patients with TSS may either have an immunodeficiency that impairs their ability to mount a humoral immune response to TSST-1 and staphylococcal enterotoxins or that the toxins inhibit the generation of an antigen-specific antibody response (see below).

3 Activation of the Immune System by TSST-1

TSST-1 does not exert direct toxic effects on the vast majority of tissues tested, even at very high concentrations (PARSONNET 1989). Rather, induction of TSS by TSST-1 may result from massive and unregulated stimulation of the immune system. In vitro tests reveal TSST-1 to be a powerful activator of lymphocytes and monocytes. TSST-1 is a potent inducer of interleukin-1 (IL-1) (IKEJIMA et al. 1984; PARSONNET et al. 1985, 1986) and tumor necrosis factor (TNF) (FAST et al. 1989; JUPIN et al. 1988; PARSONNET and GILLIS 1988) production in human monocytes, more potent on a molar basis than lipopolysaccharides (LPS). TSST-1 is also a T cell mitogen (CALVANO et al. 1984), and it induces the production of myriad T cell lymphokines including (IL-2) (CHATILA, et al. 1988; MICUSAN et al. 1986; UCHIYAMA et al. 1986), interferon-γ, lymphotoxin (TNFβ) (JUPIN et al. 1988), and colony stimulating factors (GALELLI et al. 1989). Administration of large quantities of monokines, lymphokines, or polyclonal activators of T lymphocytes to experimental animals or human subjects results in a shock state analogous to that observed with TSST-1. For example, infusion of IL-1 and TNF into rabbits reproduces the hemodynamic effects of TSST-1 infusion (IKEJIMA et al. 1989). Also, the toxicity of IL-2, administered in large quantities during treatment of cancer patients, (ROSENBERG et al. 1988) and of monoclonal antibodies directed against the T cell receptor-associated CD3 complex, administered to transplant recipients (CHATENOUD et al. 1990), is similar in many respects to the disturbances observed in patients suffering from TSS. These studies raised the possibility that the toxicity of TSST-1 is intimately related to its potent activation of immune cells.

The notion that the immunostimulatory effects of TSST-1 play an important role in the pathogenesis of TSST-1 is supported by evidence of severe histopathologic changes in the lymphoid tissues of patients with fatal TSS (PARIS et al. 1982). Lymph nodes display marked histiocytosis and hemophagocytosis in the interfollicular areas. This is frequently associated with intrafollicular or follicular lymphoid hyperplasia. Lymphoid hyperplasia is also manifest in the gastrointestinal tract, while the spleen demonstrates sinus histiocytosis and lymphoid depletion. In addition, lymphocytic infiltrates are manifest in the periportal areas of the liver and around small vessels in the skin. These findings are mirrored in rabbits inoculated with toxigenic strains of *Staphylococcus aureus* or given a constant infusion of purified TSST-1 (DE AZAVEDO et al. 1985; PARSONNET et al. 1987; RASHEED et al. 1985).

Direct proof for an obligatory role for immune cell activation in the pathogenesis of TSS has been provided by studies using immunosuppressive agents. In one study, concurrent administration of steroids together with purified TSST-1 aborted the emergence of a TSS-like illness and prevented death in four out of four rabbits tested (PARSONNET et al. 1987). In contrast, four of four rabbits receiving TSST-1 and saline died of a TSS-like illness. In another study, a murine model was developed to study the toxicity of SEB, which has also been implicated in TSS (MARRACK et al. 1990). It was demonstrated that inhibition of T lymphocyte activation with cyclosporine greatly attenuated the morbidity and mortality resulting from SEB injection in these mice.

Our understanding of the mechanism of action of TSST-1 in stimulating the immune system has been greatly clarified with the discovery that Ia molecules serve as receptors for TSST-1 (SCHOLL et al. 1989a; UCHIYAMA et al. 1989a) and that Ia-bound TSST-1 behaves as a superantigen that can stimulate large numbers of T cells in a $V_\beta 2$-specific manner (CHOI et al. 1989). TSST-1 can also act via Ia molecules to deliver growth-promoting signals to lymphocytes and to induce the production of IL-1 and TNF in monocytes. The binding of TSST-1 to Ia molecules is a property that is shared by all TSS-associated staphylococcal enterotoxins (FISCHER et al. 1989; FRASER 1989; MOLLICK et al. 1989). These toxins also behave as superantigens that activate large populations of T lymphocytes bearing distinct V_β products (CHOI et al. 1989; KAPPLER et al. 1989). Remarkably, streptococcal pyrogenic toxin A, which is related to the staphylococcal exotoxins and which has been implicated in causing a TSS-like illness (CONE et al. 1987), has also been demonstrated to bind to Ia molecules and to act as a superantigen (IMANISHI et al. 1990). These observations widen the scope of TSS to encompass a group of diseases with similar pathophysiology and clinical manifestations which are caused by Ia-binding, superantigenic, bacterial toxins.

3.1 Binding of TSST-1 to Ia Molecules

Evidence for the binding of staphylococcal exotoxins to Ia molecules was first provided by the demonstration that the mitogenic effect of these toxins is strictly dependent on the presence of Ia$^+$ accessory cells in culture, yet, unlike the case with nominal antigens, the exotoxins did not require intracellular processing (FLEISCHER and SCHREZENMEIER 1988). In the case of TSST-1, several lines of evidence were gathered indicating that this toxin binds to Ia molecules. First, TSST-1 was found to be mitogenic for peripheral blood mononuclear cells isolated from normal subjects but not from Ia-deficient patients, demonstrating a requirement for Ia$^+$ accessory cells for TSST-1 mitogenicity similar to what was found for staphylococcal enterotoxins. TSST-1 was found to bind with high affinity (K_{d50} ranging from 1.7×10^{-8} to 4.3×10^{-8}) to Ia$^+$ but not Ia$^-$ human cell lines. The number of TSST-1 binding sites per cell correlated well with Ia surface density as measured by flow cytometry. Cultured human fibroblasts, which do not constitutively express Ia molecules, failed to bind TSST-1. Induction of Ia expression on fibroblasts by treatment with interferon-γ was associated with the appearance of TSST-1 binding sites. Binding of TSST-1 to Ia$^+$ cells was inhibited by monoclonal antibodies recognizing monomorphic determinants on Ia molecules. Conclusive evidence for the binding of TSST-1 to Ia molecules was obtained by demonstrating that purified Ia molecules, but not MHC class I molecules, bind ^{125}I-labeled TSST-1 (SCHOLL and GEHA, manuscript in preparation).

TSST-1 can bind to Ia molecules of diverse isotypic and allotypic specificities. Our studies with L cells transfected with cDNAs coding for α and β chains of different Ia isotypes (DP, DQ, or DR) demonstrated that TSST-1 binds equally well and with high affinity to HLA-DR and DQ molecules (SCHOLL et al. 1990a). No detectable binding could be demonstrated for HLA-DP. However, murine L cells transfected with HLA-DP supported the proliferation of T cells in response to TSST-1, suggesting that TSST-1 does indeed bind to HLA-DP molecules but with a much lower affinity than that observed for HLA-DR or DQ molecules. These results are similar to what has been found for other staphylococcal and streptococcal superantigens, which demonstrate an affinity pattern for Ia isotypes similar to what is noted for TSST-1 (MARRACK and KAPPLER 1990). Studies on 14 different HLA-DR, 2 HLA-DQ, and 2 HLA-DP alleles demonstrated no significant difference between alleles of the same isotype in their affinity of binding to TSST-1. Also, all alleles tested were similar in their capacity to support the proliferation of human T lymphocytes in response to TSST-1. These results suggested that Ia polymorphism would play an important role in determining the response of immune cells of different individuals to TSST-1 and, consequently, the susceptibility of these individuals to TSST-1-mediated diseases. However, a different conclusion was reached in a study by Herman et al. (HERMAN et al. 1990). These authors used IL-2 production by a TSST-1-responsive murine V$_\beta$3 clone as a readout system to study the influence of isotypic and allotypic specificities of Ia molecules on the activation of T lymphocytes by TSST-1. Strong differences emerged in the abiliy of different HLA-DR allotypes to present TSST-1 to this clone. HLA-DR1 provided the best response, while HLA- DR6, DR7, and DRw53 failed to present TSST-1. This directly contrasts with the results obtained by SCHOLL et al. (1990a) in which for example, DR1 and DR7 were equally efficacious in presenting TSST-1 to human T lymphocytes. The discrepancy between the two sets of results is likely to reside in the better capacity of human TCR molecules, as compared to murine TCR molecules, to recognize TSST-1 in complex with different alleles of human Ia molecules.

In addition to binding to human Ia molecules, TSST-1 has also been demonstrated to bind to murine Ia molecules (SCHOLL et al. 1990b; UCHIYAMA et al. 1989b). However, unlike the case with human Ia molecules, the binding of TSST-1 to murine Ia molecules is governed by both isotypic and allotypic specificities. Of the two murine Ia isotypes, TSST-1 binds well to I-A but not to I-E molecules. Within I-A, allelic differences in binding to TSST-1 have been observed. Thus, TSST-1 binds well to I- A^b and to I-A^d but only weakly to I-A^k. The characteristics of TSST-1 binding to murine Ia molecules differed from those observed for other staphylococcal exotoxins such as SEA or SEB. For example, I-E molecules can support the proliferation of human T cells in response to SEA (FLEISCHER et al. 1989). These results suggest that there exist important differences between the various superantigens in their ability to bind murine Ia molecules.

Superantigens bind to a site on Ia molecules outside of the antigen groove. Extensive mutations of Ia $\alpha 1$ residues that form one face of the antigen groove fail to affect the presentation of superantigens to T cells (DELLABONA et al. 1990). In contrast, the same mutations drastically affect the ability of Ia molecules to present nominal antigen to T cells. A similar conclusion was reached in another study on the binding of TSST-1 to Ia molecules, which failed to document an effect of TSST-1 on the binding of antigenic peptides to Ia molecules (KARP et al. 1990). The same study took advantage of the disparity in the affinity of binding of TSST-1 to HLA-DR vs HLA-DP molecules to map the binding site of TSST-1 on Ia molecules. A series of chimeric HLA DR/HLA DP molecules were generated and expressed in L cells, in which part of the sequence of either the α or the β chain was substituted by the corresponding sequence of the heterologous isotype. Thus, DR α chains that were paired with DR/DP β chains bound [125]I- labeled TSST-1, whereas DP α chains that were paired with DP/DR β chains did not. This suggested that it is the α chain that determines the efficacy of binding of TSST-1 to Ia molecules. Furthermore, substituting the $\alpha 2$ domain of HLA-DR α chain with that of HLA-DP did not diminish the binding of TSST-1, indicating that it is the $\alpha 1$ domain that is critical for binding of TSST-1 to Ia molecules. Another approach for mapping the binding site of TSST-1 to Ia molecules took advantage of the binding of TSST-1 to HLA-DR molecules but not to the highly homologous murine I-E molecules. L cell transfectants expressing hybrid DRα:I-Eβ, **but not I-Eα- DR1β molecules,** could bind ^{125}I-labeled TSST-1 (SCHOLL et al. 1990b). This suggested that it is the α chain specificity that is critical for the binding of TSST-1 to Ia molecules, in agreement with the results obtained using HLA-DR/DP hybrid molecules.

Different superantigens may bind to different sites on Ia molecules (SCHOLL et al. 1989b). This has been most clearly demonstrated for TSST-1 and SEB. Neither toxin is capable of displacing the binding of the other toxin to B cell lines or to L cells transfected with Ia molecules. The capacity of murine I-E molecules to support SEA-but not TSST-1-induced mitogenesis also argues for strong differences between TSST-1 and other toxins in their binding to Ia molecules.

The sites within TSST-1 responsible for binding to Ia molecules have not yet been mapped; however, there are clues as to their location. TSST-1 is a 22 kDa protein composed of 194 amino acids (BLOMSTER-HAUTAMAA et al. 1986a). Previous studies using cyanogen bromide-generated fragments revealed that monoclonal antibodies that inhibited toxin-induced T cell proliferation reacted with a 14–15 kDa internal fragment (BLOMSTER-HAUTAMAA et al. 1986b; KOKAN-MOORE and BERGDOLL 1989). Further studies identified one epitope, a ten amino acid stretch spanning residues 34–43, that is recognized by a neutralizing monoclonal antibody (MURPHY et al. 1988). Additional information was provided by studies on toxin fragments generated using the protease papain. Biological activity, as assayed by mitogenicity and by reactivity to neutralizing anti-TSST-1 monoclonal antibodies, was maintained in a 12 kDa peptide spanning residues 88–194 of the toxin (EDWIN et al. 1988). It is reasonable to assume that this stretch contains both the Ia binding site and the site interacting with V_β residues on the T cell receptor and that additional site(s) at the N-terminal region of the molecule may regulate the conformation of the molecule and provide sites for some neutralizing antibodies. Studies with overlapping peptides spanning the entire TSST-1 sequence at 20 amino acid stretches at a time have demonstrated that no one peptide can either inhibit or mimic the binding of TSST-1 to Ia molecules (RAMESH and GEHA, unpublished observations). This suggested that the Ia binding site may be formed by a complex three- dimensional epitope not reproduced by any of the studied peptides.

3.2 Functional Consequences of Toxin/Ia Interaction

The binding of TSST-1 to Ia molecules initiates the activation of diverse immune cells including T and B lymphocytes, monocytes, and natural killer (NK) cells. Two major mechanisms account for the activation of immune cells by TSST-1. The first mechanism accounts for the activation of T lymphocytes by TSST-1 and involves the engagement of the V_β component of the T cell receptor by toxin/Ia complexes resulting in T cell activation and proliferation. The second mechanism involves the transduction via Ia molecules of signals that result in the activation of Ia$^+$ immune cells including B lymphocytes, monocytes, activated NK cells, and activated T lymphocytes.

3.2.1 Activation of T Lymphocytes

The mitogenic effect of TSST-1 is strictly dependent on the presence of Ia$^+$ accessory cells. Radioligand binding assays fail to demonstrate binding of TSST-1 to Ia$^-$ T lymphocytes. Also, unlike the case of mitogenic anti-T cell receptor antibodies, TSST-1 is not mitogenic when cross-linked on plastic and presented to T lymphocytes in the presence of IL-2. Interestingly, purified Ia molecules cross-linked on plastic can support the proliferation of T lymphocytes in response to TSST-1 and IL-2 (SCHOLL and GEHA, manuscript in preparation). These results indicate that a specific high-affinity interaction between TSST-1 and T cell receptor molecules first requires the binding of TSST-1 to Ia molecules.

In the presence of Ia$^+$ accessory cells, TSST-1 induces the proliferative of T cells and the production of large quantities of lymphokines. However, not all T cells in culture respond to TSST-1. The uneven proliferative responses of different T cells to TSST-1 can be readily demonstrated using T cell clones, some of which respond vigorously to TSST-1 while others fail to do so. The clonal variability between T cells in their mitogenic response to TSST-1 and other superantigens has been determined to be governed by the V_β specificity of the responding T lymphocytes. In the case of TSST-1, only those lymphocytes expressing $V_\beta 2$ proliferate in response to TSST-1. This has been demonstrated to be true both in vitro, where treatment of peripheral blood mononuclear cells with TSST-1 results in the selective expansion of $V_\beta 2$-expressing T cells, and in vivo, where patients with TSS demonstrate massive expansion of their $V_\beta 2 +$ T lymphocyte population (CHOI et al. 1990b). TSST-1 can also activate murine T cells in a V_β-restricted manner (MARRACK and KAPPLER 1990). Murine T lymphocytes activated by TSST-1 include those bearing $V_\beta 3$, $V_\beta 15$, and $V_\beta 17$ products.

The molecular interactions governing the recognition of TSST-1/Ia complexes by $V_\beta 2$-compatible T cell receptor molecules have not been specifically addressed. They may, however, be similar to what has been described for another staphylococcal enterotoxin, staphylococcal enterotoxin C2 (SEC2) (CHOI et al. 1990a). SEC2/Ia complexes were recognized by chimeric murine T cell receptor molecules bearing human $V_\beta 13.2$, but not $V_\beta 13.1$, product. This confirmed the permissive role of the T cell receptor α chain in the interaction of the β chain with toxin/Ia complexes. Further studies identified the V_β specificity of this toxin to be governed by a single stretch of eight amino acids facing away from the peptide antigen/Ia binding site and found in $V_\beta 13.2$ but not in $V_\beta 13.1$. The interaction between TSST-1 and the T cell receptor β chain is contributed to by an additional interaction between the T cell receptor and Ia molecules. This is supported by findings discussed in the previous section and demonstrating that TSST-1, bound by the same DR allele, e.g., DR7, is recognized by human but not by murine V_β-compatible T lymphocytes. The site on TSST-1 recognized by the T cell receptor is not known, but it clearly localizes to the distal two-thirds of the molecule, as this portion of TSST-1 is fully mitogenic. The inability to demonstrate an interaction between the T cell receptor and TSST-1 in the absence of Ia molecules suggests that the epitope on TSST-1 recognized by the T cell receptor results from a conformational change in the toxin molecule that takes place upon its binding to Ia molecules.

Ia-bound TSST-1 activates both CD4$^+$ and CD8$^+$ T lymphocytes (CALVANO et al. 1984), in marked distinction to Ia-bound nominal antigens which activate CD4$^+$ cells only. The role of CD4 in the interaction of TSST-1/Ia complex with T cell receptor molecules was examined using CD4$^-$ murine T cell hybridomas. Induction of CD4 expression by transfection with retroviral vectors containing CD4 cDNA did not affect the proliferative response of the majority of these hybridomas to TSST-1 or ot other bacterial superantigens, indicating that CD4 is not required for the interaction between TSST-1/Ia complexes and T cell receptor molecules. This may reflect the high-affinity nature of TSST-1/Ia/TCR interaction, as CD4 expression is required in cases of low-affinity, but not high-affinity, interactions between nominal antigen Ia complexes and TCR molecules (MARRACK et al. 1983).

Engagement of $V_\beta 2$ by TSST-1/Ia complexes results in the initiation of early activation events similar to those observed upon engagement of the T cell receptor with nominal antigen/Ia complexes or with anti-T cell receptor antibodies (CHATILA et al. 1988; NORTON et al. 1990). These include the activation of T cell receptor-coupled phospholipase C. This enzyme hydrolyzes membrane phosphoinositides to generate second messengers such as diacylglycerol, which activates protein kinase C, and inositol phosphates, which effect a rise in the free intracellular Ca^{+2} concentration. These early activation events are thought to mediate both the induction of lymphokine and lymphokine receptor gene expression and the progression of T cells through the cell cycle.

Ia molecules expressed on TSST-1-activated T lymphocytes can initiate further cycles of T cell activation and proliferation by presenting TSST-1 to T cell receptor molecules. This has been demonstrated using Ia$^+$ T cell clones bearing the appropriate V_β product, which proliferate vigorously in response to TSST-1 in the absence of any added accessory cells (SPERTINI et al. 1991). TSST-1 can be presented to T cell receptor molecules by Ia molecules found on the same lymphocyte (cis presentation) or by Ia molecules present on other T lymphocytes (trans presentation). The induction by TSST-1 of sustained Ca^{+2} mobilization in these lymphocytes within seconds after its addition despite constant stirring suggests that cis presentation may be the dominant mechanism involved.

Recently, we have elucidated another mechanism that can help perpetuate the activation of T lymphocytes by TSST-1. This involves the delivery of trophic signals via Ia molecules that are expressed on activated T lymphocytes and which results in the activation and proliferation of these lymphocytes in a V_β unrestricted manner (SPERTINI et al. 1991). This has been demonstrated using Ia$^+$ T cell clones bearing a mismatched V_β product. Unlike the V_β-matched T cell clones, the mismatched clones fail to proliferate in response to TSST-1 in the absence of accessory cells. However, they proliferate vigorously in response to TSST-1 in the presence of either Ia$^+$ or Ia$^-$ accessory cells, suggesting that the activation signal is delivered via Ia molecules on T lymphocytes and requires an Ia-independent accessory cell signal. Further evidence for this scheme has been obtained using T cell clones derived from Ia$^-$ deficient patients and lacking any detectable surface expression of Ia molecules. Unlike Ia$^+$ T cell clones, Ia$^-$ clones proliferate to TSST-1 only in a V_β-restricted manner. This indicated that the proliferation of Ia$^-$ clones can only be achieved by cognate interaction between Ia/toxin molecules on accessory cells and $V_\beta 2^+$ T cell receptor molecules on T lymphocytes.

3.2.2 Activation of B Lymphocytes

B lymphocytes express Ia molecules throughout much of their development and differentiation and are thus targets of TSST-1 binding and action. Postmortem studies on lymph nodes of patients with fatal TSS revealed evidence of both follicular and intrafollicular hyperplasia, suggesting in vivo activation and proliferation of follicular B lymphocytes. In vitro studies reveal that by itself TSST-1 does not cause the proliferation of B lymphocytes or their differentiation into immunoglobulin (Ig)-producing cells. However, in the presence of T lymphocytes, TSST-1 induces intense proliferation of B lymphocytes and promotes their differentiation into Ig-secreting lymphocytes (MOURAD et al. 1989). TSST-1-inducing Ig production is critically dependent on the presence of an optimal load of T lymphocytes in culture with B lymphocytes, estimated at a 1:20 ratio of T to B lymphocytes. Interestingly, this ratio corresponds to the ratio of T to B lymphocytes normally found in lymph node follicles (HEINEN et al. 1988). Higher T lymphocyte loads result in a progressive decline in TSST-1-induced Ig production. This may help explain the observation that TSST-1 inhibits both spontaneous and pokeweed mitogen- induced Ig production in unfractionated peripheral blood mononuclear cells. It is possible that inhibitory T/B cell interactions dominate at higher T cell loads. Alternatively, massive activation of large numbers of T lymphocytes by TSST-1 may result in the attainment of a critical concentration of cytokine(s) inhibitory for TSST-1-triggered Ig production.

The mechanism by which TSST-1 induces T lymphocyte-dependent B lymphocyte proliferation and Ig production resides in its capacity to mediate cognate interaction between B lymphocytes and T lymphocytes. This interaction mimics the interaction between antigen presenting B lymphocytes and antigen responding T lymphocytes in its requirement for the participation of Ia molecules, T cell receptor/CD3 complexes, and adhesion molecules, especially LFA-1 and its counter receptors. TSST-1 does not require the participation of CD4 molecules in its mediation of cognate interaction between T and B lymphocytes. As discussed in the previous section, this may reflect the high-affinity nature of the interaction between the Ia/toxin complex and the TCR/CD3 complex, as CD4 functions to bolster low-affinity, but not high-affinity, antigen-TCR interactions. Another distinction betwen antigen and TSST-1-triggered T/B cell interactions is that the latter is not restricted to a particular Ia allele and can proceed between Ia mismatched T and B lymphocytes. The ability of TSST-1 to mediate Ia-unrestricted cognate interaction between large numbers of unprimed T and B cells provides a useful model for the study of antigen-driven, T lymphocyte-dependent, B lymphocyte proliferation and Ig production.

Polyclonal activation of B lymphocytes by TSST-1 can result in the inhibition of humoral immune responses to nominal antigens, including TSST-1 itself. This may explain the inability of many TSS patients to mount an antibody response to TSST-1. As discussed earlier in this review, the majority of patients lack antibodies to TSST-1 on their first presentation with TSS, suggesting that they have not previously encountered TSST-1 as a nominal antigen. The consequent polyclonal T and B lymphocyte activation may prevent them from mounting such a humoral immune response, making them susceptible to recurrent TSS. Supporting evidence for such a scenario has been provided by studies on a murine model of enterotoxin toxicity, in which mice exhibited severely defective immune response to a nominal antigen administered simultaneously with SEB.

While TSST-1 does not on its own induce the proliferation or differentiation of purified B lymphocytes, it does deliver activation signals to B lymphocytes via Ia molecules. TSST-1 synergizes with B cell mitogens such as phorbol myristate acetate (PMA) or anti-surface Ig antibodies in inducing the proliferation of B lymphocytes (FULEIHAN et al. 1991). Further evidence for signal transduction via Ia molecules in B lymphocytes has been provided by the demonstration that both TSST-1 and monoclonal antibodies that recognize an epitope closely related to the TSST-1 binding site on Ia molecules induce sustained LFA-1 dependent adhesion (MOURAD et al. 1990). This adhesion was effected by the activation of LFA-1 adhesion function and not that of its counter receptors. Induction of cell adhesion by TSST-1 was also observed in Ia$^+$ T lymphocytes and monocytes and Ia$^+$, but not Ia$^-$, B lymphoblastoid cell lines. This suggested that adhesion induced via Ia reflects a function common to Ia molecules in diverse cell types (see below).

3.2.3 Activation of NK Cells

Resting NK cells do not express Ia molecules on their surface and are thus not a target for TSST-1 action. Nevertheless, these cells, which constitutively express IL-2 receptors, can be potentially activated by IL-2 produced by TSST-1-activated T lymphocytes. Another mechanism for NK cell activation can proceed by the induction of Ia expression by another lymphokine produced by TSST-1-activated T lymphocytes, namely, interferon-γ. TSST-1 can then bind to and directly induce the proliferation of such Ia$^+$ NK cells. This has been demonstrated using Ia$^+$, CD56$^+$, CD3$^-$ NK clones (SPERTINI et al. 1991). TSST-1-induced proliferation of NK clones proceeded in the absence of accessory cells but was enhanced upon the addition of accessory cells to cultures. It was inhibited by anti-Ia monoclonal antibodies that block the binding of TSST-1 to Ia molecules. These results suggested that TSST-1 induced proliferation of NK clones was triggered by signaling via Ia molecules.

3.2.4 Induction of Monokine Synthesis

The similarity between TSST-1-mediated toxic shock and endotoxin-mediated shock led investigators soon after the discovery of TSST-1 to examine whether it can mimic endotoxin in inducing IL-1 synthesis. It was quickly appreciated that TSST-1 is a potent inducer of IL-1 synthesis, more potent on a molar basis than endotoxin (IKEJIMA et al. 1984; PARSONNET et al. 1985, 1986). Later, TSST-1 was also demonstrated to induce the synthesis of TNF in human monocytes (FAST et al. 1989; JUPIN et al. 1988; PARSONNET and GILLIS 1988). Induction of IL-1 and TNF synthesis by TSST-1 does not require the presence of T lymphocytes as can be demonstrated in TSST-1-treated monocytic cell lines (HIROSE et al. 1985). The presence of T lymphocytes may, however, enhance the efficacy of TSST-1 in inducing monokine synthesis (FISCHER et al. 1990). We have recently demonstrated that induction of IL-1 and TNF synthesis by TSST-1 is effected by transcriptional activation of the respective monokine gene, resulting in a dramatic increase in the level of newly initiated monokine RNA molecules and in monokine mRNA steady state levels in the nuclei and cytosol of stimulated monocytic cells, respectively (TREDE et al. 1991). Monokine mRNA species are first detected within 30 min after TSST-1 treatment; their levels peak at 3 h poststimulation and decline thereafter. Transcriptional activation of monokine genes by TSST-1 does not require prior protein synthesis as it proceeds in monocytes pretreated with cycloheximide, an inhibitor of protein synthesis. Monoclonal antibodies that recognize epitopes closely related to the TSST-1 binding site on Ia molecules also induce monokine mRNA accumulation. This is in agreement with previous reports demonstrating that some anti-Ia monoclonal antibodies induce IL-1 synthesis (PALACIOS 1985; PALKAMA et al. 1989) and indicates that TSST-1 transduces activation signals via Ia molecules that result in the induction of monokine gene transcription.

4 Mechanisms of Signal Transduction via Ia Molecules by TSST-1

Insight into the nature of activation signals transduced by TSST-1 via Ia was first gained by studying Ia-mediated induction of cell adhesion. It was demonstrated that adhesion induced by TSST-1 and other Ia ligands was reversed by the protein kinase C-specific inhibitor sphinghosine but not by its inert metabolite ceramide (MOURAD et al. 1990). This suggested that the binding of TSST-1 to Ia molecules induced intracellular activation signals that resulted in protein kinase C activation and consequent up-regulation of LFA-1 adhesion function.

Further insight into signaling by TSST-1 via Ia molecules was provided by studying the role of protein kinases in the induction of monokine gene expression by TSST-1 using protein kinase inhibitors. Treatment of monocytes with the protein kinase C inhibitors sphingosine and H7 or the tyrosine kinase inhibitor genistein inhibited the induction of monokine gene expression by TSST-1. In contrast, inhibitors of cAMP-dependent protein kinases such as HA1004 did not affect the accumulation of IL-1 and TNF mRNA induced by TSST-1 (TREDE et al., manuscript in preparation). These results suggested that transcriptional activation of monokine genes by TSST-1 is mediated by the activation of protein kinase C and of protein tyrosine kinase(s), acting either in series or in parallel. Activation of protein kinase C and tyrosine kinase(s) by TSST-1 echoes the activation of these kinases via lymphocyte antigen receptors (ASHWELL and KLAUSNER 1990) and receptors for growth factors (ULLRICH and SCHLESSINGER 1990) and suggests that signaling via Ia molecules shares common features with signaling via the aforementioned receptors.

Transcriptional activation of cytokine genes is mediated by a set of DNA binding factors that recognize distinct regulatory sequences found within the promotor and enhancer regions of these genes (CRABTREE 1989). Examination of IL-1β (CLARK et al. 1986), TNFα, and TNFβ (NEDOSPASOV et al. 1986) genomic sequences reveals DNA sequences recognized by AP-1, AP-2, and NF-κB DNA binding proteins. These factors mediate the transcriptional activation of many genes by activators of protein kinase C such as PMA, which itself is a potent inducer of IL-1 and TNF gene transcription. Prior treatment of monocytic cells with cycloheximide does not affect the transcriptional activation of monokine genes by LPS or by PMA (FENTON et al. 1988). This makes it unlikely that inducible nuclear binding factors such as AP-1 mediate the transcriptional activation of monokine genes by LPS and PMA and suggests instead a role for constitutively expressed DNA binding proteins such as NF-κB in mediating this effect. Direct evidence for a role for NF-κB in the activation of murine TNFα gene transcription by LPS has been recently provided in a study by SHAKHOV et al.(1990), who demonstrated two NF-κB sites in the TNFα 5' region critical for responsiveness to LPS. Transcriptional activation of monokine genes by TSST-1 is similar to that induced by LPS both in its time course and its independence of de novo protein synthesis. This would argue for a role for NF-κB in the induction of monokine gene transcription by Ia ligands. Studies are currently under way to verify this possibility.

5 TSS and Endotoxin-Mediated Shock: Common and Divergent Pathogenic Mechanisms

As alluded to previously, the pathophysiology of TSS bears resemblance to LPS-mediated gram-negative bacterial sepsis. In each of these conditions, the pathogenic bacterial product induces the release of monokines such as IL-1 and TNF implicated in causing tissue injury. Induction of monokine synthesis by TSST-1 and LPS may proceed via a common mechanism, with LPS activating intracellular signaling mechanisms normally coupled to Ia molecules and amenable to activation by extracellular ligands such as TSST-1. IL-1 (OKUSAWA et al. 1988) and TNF (TRACEY et al. 1986) precipitate shock when infused into experimental animals, and the combination of both monokines exhibits synergisim in inducing shock (IKEJIMA et al. 1989; OKUSAWA et al. 1988). Conversely, anti-TNF antibodies protect experimental animals from endotoxin-mediated shock (TRACEY et al. 1987). It is thus likely that monokine release helps mediate the shock state observed in both conditions. However, unlike endotoxin-mediated sepsis, TSS is additionally associated with the activation of a significant portion of T lymphocytes as a result of superantigen-mediated activation by TSST-1 and related toxins. The consequent outpouring of lymphokines may synergize with monokines to aggravate the shock state.

Activated lymphocytes with enhanced adhesive properties may interact with vascular endothelium to induce inflammation, end organ damage, and vascular permeability. The ability of different staphylococcal exotoxins to activate populations of T cells bearing distinct V_β products would result in an even greater degree of T cell activation by staphylococcal isolates producing multiple toxins. Such isolates may be associated with a higher fatality rate, as has been observed for those isolates producing TSST-1 and SEC1 (CRASS and BERGDOLL 1986). T lymphocyte activation may also account for some of the peculiar manifestations of TSS such as the generalized erythroderma, a condition that may reflect intense lymphocyte activation and infiltration around small blood vessels in the skin, and periportal lymphocytic infiltration in the liver. The powerful effecs of TSST-1 on the immune system may account for the tenacity of the shock state that is observed in other wise young and healthy individuals and which is mediated at times by very small pockets of staphylococcal infection.

6 Future Directions

The discovery that TSST-1 serves as an Ia-binding superantigen has greatly clarified the mechanisms by which this and other related staphylococcal exotoxins induce TSS. This will hopefully allow the development of rational strategies for countering the effects of TSST-1 on the immune system, including the design of peptides that interfere with the binding of toxin to Ia molecules. The ready availability of TSST-1 as a high-affinity agonistic Ia ligand provides a tool that can help unravel transmembrane signaling processes via Ia molecules. This will greatly expand our information on this important receptor system and the role it plays in the course of a normal immune response and in disease states.

References

Ashwell JD, Klausner RD (1990) Genetic and mutational analysis of the T cell antigen receptor. Annu Rev Immunol 8: 139–168

Bergdoll MS, Crass BA, Reiser RF, Robbins RN, Davis JP (1981) A new staphylococcal enterotoxin, enterotoxin F, associated with toxic shock syndrome staphylococcal aureus isolates. Lancet 1: 1017–1021

Best GK, Scott DF, Kling JM, Thompson MR, Adinolfi LE, Bonventre PF (1988) Protection of rabbits in an infection model of toxic shock syndrome by a TSS toxin-1-specific monoclonal antibody. Infect Immun 56: 998–999

Blomster-Hautamaa DA, Kreiswirth BN, Kornblum JS, Novick RP, Schlievert PM (1986a) The nucleotide and partial amino acid sequence of toxic shock syndrome toxin-1. J Biol Chem 261: 15783–15786

Blomster-Hautamaa DA, Novick RP, Schlievert PM (1986b) Localization of biological function of toxic shock syndrome toxin-1 by use of monoclonal antibodies and cyanogen bromide generated toxin fragment. J Immunol 137: 3572–3576

Bonventre PF, Thompson MR, Adinolfi LE, Gillis ZA, Parsonet J (1988) Neutralization of toxic shock syndrome toxin-1 by monoclonal antibodies in vitro and in vivo. Infect Immun 56: 135–141

Bonventre PF, Wekbach L, Harth G, Haidaris C (1989) Distribution and expression of toxic shock syndrome toxin-1 gene among staphylococcal aureus isolates of toxin shock syndrome and non-toxic shock syndrome origin. Rev Infect Dis [Suppl 1] 11: S90–S95

Calvano SE, Quimby FW, Antonacci AC, Reiser RF, Bergdoll MS, Dineen P (1984) Analysis of the mitogenic effects of toxic shock toxin on human peripheral blood mononuclear cells in vitro. Clin Immunol Immunopathol 33: 99–110

Chatenoud L, Ferran C, Legendre C, Thouard I, Merite S, Reuter A, Gevaert Y, Kreis H, Franchimont P, Bach JF (1990) In vivo cell activation following OKT3 administration. Systemic cytokine release and modulation by corticosteroids. Transplantation 49: 697–702

Chatila T, Wood N, Parsonnet J, Geha RS (1988) Toxic shock syndrome toxin-1 induces inositol phospholipid turnover, protein kinase C translocation, and calcium mobilization in human T cells. J Immunol 140: 1250–1255

Chesney PJ (1989) Clinical aspects and spectrum of illness of toxic shock syndrome: overview. Rev Infect Dis [Supp 1] 11: S1–S7

Choi Y, Kotzin B, Herron L, Callahan J, Marrack P, Kappler J (1989) Interaction of *Staphylococcus aureus* toxin superantigens with human T cells. Proc Natl Acad Sci USA 86: 8941–8945

Choi Y, Herman A, DiGiusto D, Wade T, Marrack P, Kappler J (1990a) Residues of the variable region of the T cell receptor β chain that interact with *S. aureus* toxin superantigens. Nature 346: 471–473

Choi Y, Lafferty JA, Clements JR, Todd JK, Gelfand EW, Kappler J, Marrack P, Kotzin BL (1990b) Selective expansion of T cells expressing Vβ2 in toxic shock syndrome. J Exp Med 172: 981–984

Clark BD, Collins KL, Gandy MS, Webb AC, Auron PE (1986) Genomic sequence for human prointerleukin-1 beta: possible evolution from a reverse transcribed prointerleukin-1 alpha gene. Nucleic Acids Res 14: 7897–7914

Cone LA, Woodward DR, Schlievert PM, Tomory GS (1987) Clinical and bacteriological observations of a toxic shock-like syndrome due to *Streptococcus pyogenes*. N Engl J Med 317: 146–149

Crabtree G (1989) Contingent genetic regulatory events in T lymphocytes. Science 243: 355–361

Crass BA, Bergdoll MS (1986) Toxin involvement in toxic shock syndrome. J Infect Dis 153: 918–926

Davis JP, Chesney PJ, Wand PJ, LaVenture M (1980) Toxic-shock syndrome: epidemiological features, recurrence, risk factors and prevention. N Engl J Med 303: 1429–1435

De Azavedo JCS, Foster TJ, Hartigan PJ, Arbuthnott JP, O'Reilly M, Kreiswirth BN, Novick RP (1985) Expression of the cloned toxic shock syndrome toxin-1 gene (tst) in vivo with a rabbit uterine model. Infect Immun 50: 304–309

Dellabona P, Peccoud J, Kappler J, Marrack P, Benoist C, Mathis D (1990) Superantigens interact with MHC class II molecules outside of the antigen groove. Cell 62: 1115–1121

Edwin C, Parsonnet J, Kass EH (1988) Structure-activity relationship of toxic shock syndrome toxin-1: derivation and characterization of immunologically and biologically active fragments. J Infect Dis 158: 1287–1295

Fast DJ, Schlievert PM, Nelson RD (1989) Toxic shock syndrome-associated staphylococcal and streptococcal pyrogenic toxins are potent inducers of tumor necrosis factor production. Infect Immun 57: 291–294

Fenton MJ, Vermeulin MW, Clark BD, Webb AC, Auron PE (1988) Human pro-IL-1β gene expression in monocytic cells is regulated by two distinct pathways. J Immunol 140: 2267–2273

Fischer H, Dohlsten M, Lindvall M, Sjögren H-O, Carlsson R (1989) Binding of staphylococcal enterotoxin A to HLA-DR on B cell lines. J Immunol 142(9): 3151–3157

Fischer H, Dohlsten M, Anderson U, Hedlund G, Ericson P, Hanson J, Sjögren HO (1990) Production of TNF-α and TNF-β by staphylococcal enterotoxin A activated human T cells. J Immunol 144: 4663–4669

Fleischer B, Schrezenmeier H (1988) T cell stimulation by staphylococcal enterotoxins. J Exp Med 167: 1697–1707

Fleischer B, Schrezenmeier H, Conradt P (1989) T lymphocyte activation by staphylococcal enterotoxins: role of class II molecules and T cell surface structures. Cell Immunol 120: 92–101

Fraser JD (1989) High-affinity binding of staphylococcal enterotoxins A and B to HLA-DR. Nature 339: 221–223

Fuleihan R, Mourad W, Geha RS, Chatila T (1991) Engagement of MHC-class II molecules by the staphylococcal exotoxin TSST-1 delivers a progression signal to mitogen activated B cells. J Immunol (in press)

Galelli A, Anderson S, Charlot B, Alouf JE (1989) Induction of murine hemopoietic growth factors by toxic shock syndrome toxin-1. J Immunol 142: 2855–2863

Heinen E, Cormann N, Kinet-Denoel C (1989) The lymph follicle: a hard nut to crack. Immunol Today 9: 240–243

Herman A, Crotreau G, Sekaly R-P, Kappler J, Marrack P (1990) HLA-DR alleles differ in their ability to present staphyococcal enterotoxins to T cells. J Exp Med 172: 709–717

Hirose A, Ikejima T, Gill M (1985) Established macrophage-like cell lines synthesize interleukin-1 in response to toxic shock syndrome toxin. Infect Immun 50: 765–770

Ikejima T, Dinarello CA, Gill DM, Wolff SM (1984) Induction of human interleukin-1 by a product of *Staphylococcus aureus* associated with toxic shock syndrome. J Clin Invest 73: 1312–1320

Ikejima T, Okusawa S, van der Meer WM, Dinarello CA (1989) Toxic shock syndrome is mediated by interleukin-1 and tumor necrosis factor. Rev Infect Dis [Suppl 1] 11: S316–S317

Imanishi K, Igarashi H, Uchiyama T (1990) Activation of murine T cells by streptococcal pyrogenic exotoxin type A: requirement for MHC class II molecules on accessory cells and identification of Vβ elements in T cell receptor of toxin-reactive T cells. J Immunol 145: 3170–3176

Jupin C, Anderson S, Damais C, Alouf J (1988) Toxic shock syndrome toxin-1 as an inducer of human tumor necrosis factor and γ interferon. J Exp Med 167: 752–761

Kappler J, Kotzin B, Herron L, Gelfand EW, Bigler RD, Boylston A, Carrel S, Posnett DN, Choi Y, Marrack P (1989) Vβ-specific stimulation of human T cell by staphylococcal toxins. Science 244: 811–813

Karp DR, Teletski CL, Scholl P, Geha R, Long EO (1990) The α1 domain of the HLA-DR molecule is essential for high-affinity binding of the toxic shock syndrome toxin-1. Nature 346: 474–476

Kokan-Moore NP, Bergdoll MS (1989) Determination of the biologically active region in toxic shock syndrome toxin-1. Rev Infect Dis [Suppl 1] 11: S125–S1296

Marrack P, Kappler J (1990) The staphylococcal enterotoxins and their relatives. Science 248: 705–711

Marrack P, Ender R, Shimonkevitz R, Zlotnik A, Dialynas D, Fitch F, Kappler J (1983) The major histocompatibility complex-restricted antigen receptor on T cells. II. Role of the L3T4 product. J Exp Med 158: 1077–1091

Marrack P, Blackman M, Kushner E, Kappler J (1990) The toxicity of staphylococcal enterotoxin B in mice is mediated by T cells. J Exp Med 171: 455–464

Micusan VV, Mercier G, Bahtti AR, Reiser RF, Bergdoll MS (1986) Production of human and murine interleukin-2 by toxic shock syndrome toxin-1. Immunology 58: 203–207

Mollick JA, Cook RG, Rich RR (1989) Class II MHC molecules are specific receptors for staphylococcus enterotoxin A. Science 244: 817–820

Mourad W, Scholl P, Diez A, Geha R, Chatila T (1989) The staphylococcal toxin TSST-1 triggers B cell proliferation and differentiation via MHC unrestricted cognate T/B cell interaction. J Exp Med 170: 2011–2022

Mourad W, Geha RS, Chatila T (1990) Engagement of major histocompatibility complex class II molecules induces sustained, LFA-1 dependent cell adhesion. J Exp Med 172: 1513–1516

Murphy BG, Kreiswirth BN, Novick RP, Schlievert PM (1988) Localization of a biologically important epitope on toxic shock syndrome toxin-1. J Infect Dis 158: 549–555

Nedospasov SA, Shakov AN, Turetskaya RL, Mett VA, Azizov MM, Georgiev GP, Korobko VG, Dobrynin VN, Filippov SA, Bystrov NS, Boldyreva EF, Chuvpilo SA, Chumakov AM, Ovchinnikov YA (1986) Tandem arrangement of genes coding for tumor necrosis factor (TNF-α) and lymphotoxin (TNF-β) in the human genome. Cold Spring Harbor Symp Quant Biol 511: 611

Norton SD, Schliveret PM, Novick RP, Jenkins MK (1990) Molecular requirements for T cell activation by the staphylococcal toxic shock syndrome toxin-1. J Immunol 144: 2089–2095

Okusawa S, Gelfand JA, Ikejima T, Connolly RJ, Dinarello CA (1988) Interleukin 1 induces a shock-like state in rabbits. Synergism with tumor necrosis factor and the effect of cyclooxygenase inhibition. J Clin Invest 81: 1162–1172

Palacios R (1985) Monoclonal antibodies against human Ia antigens stimulate monocytes to secrete interleukin 1. Proc Natl Acad Sci USA 82: 6652–6656

Palkama T, Sihvola M, Hurme M (1989) Induction of interleukin 1α (IL-1α) and IL-1β mRNA expression and cellular IL-1 production by anti-HLA-DR antibodies in human monocytes. Scand J Immunol 29: 609–615

Paris AL, Herwaldt LA, Blum D, Schmid GP, Shands KN, Broome CV (1982) Pathologic findings in twelve fatal cases of toxic shock syndrome. Ann Intern Med 96: 852–857

Parsonnet J (1989) Mediators in the pathogenesis of toxic shock syndrome: an overview. Rev Infect Dis [Suppl 1] 11: S263–S269

Parsonnet J, Gillis ZA (1988) Production of tumor necrosis factor by human monocytes in response to toxic shock syndrome toxin-1. J Infect Dis 158: 1026–1033

Parsonnet J, Gillis ZA, Pier GB (1986) Induction of interleukin-1 by strains of Staphylococcus aureus from patients with nonmenstrual toxic shock syndrome. J Infect Dis 154: 55–63

Parsonnet J, Hickman RK, Eardley DP, Pier GB (1985) Induction of human interleukin-1 by toxic shock syndrome toxin-1. J Infect Dis 151: 514–522

Parsonnet J, Gillis ZA, Richter AG, Pier GB (1987) A rabbit model of toxic shock syndrome that uses a constant, subcutaneous infusion of toxic shock syndrome toxin-1. Infect Immun 55: 1070–1076

Rasheed JK, Arko RJ, Feely JC, Chandler FW, Thornsberry C, Gibson RJ, Cohen ML, Jeffries CD, Broome CV (1985) Acquired ability of Staphylococcus aureus to produce toxic shock associated protein and resulting illness in a rabbit model. Infect Immun 47: 598–604

Rosenberg SA, Lotze MT, Mule JJ (1988) New approaches to the immunotherapy of cancer using interleukin-2. Ann Intern Med 108: 853–864

Schlievert PM (1986) Staphylococcal enterotoxin B and toxic-shock syndrome toxin-1 are significantly associated with non-menstrual TSS (Letter). Lancet 1: 1149–1150

Schlievert PM, Shands KN, Dan BB, Schmid GP, Nishimura RD (1981) Identification and characterization of an exotoxin from Staphylococcus aureus associated with toxic shock syndrome. J Infect Dis 143: 509–516

Scholl P, Diez A, Mourad W, Parsonnet J, Geha RS, Chatila T (1989a) Toxic shock syndrome toxin-1 binds to class II major histocompatibility molecules. Proc Natl Acad Sci USA 86: 4210–4214

Scholl PR, Diez A, Geha RS (1989b) Staphylococcal enterotoxin B and toxic shock syndrome toxin-1 bind to distinct sites on HLA-DR and HLA-DQ molecules. J Immunol 143: 2583

Scholl PR, Diez A, Karr R, Sekaly RP, Trowsdale J, Geha RS (1990a) Effects of isotypes and allelic polymorphism on the binding of staphylococcal exotoxins to MHC class II molecules. J Immunol 144: 226–230

Scholl PR, Diez A, Sekaly RP, Glimcher L, Geha RS (1990b) Binding of toxic shock syndrome toxin-1 to murine MHC class II molecules. Eur J Immunol 20: 1911–1916

Shakhov AN, Collart MA, Vassalli P, Nedospasov SA, Jongeneel CV (1990) kB-type enhancers are involved in lipopolysaccharide-mediated transcriptional activation of the tumor necrosis factor a gene in primary macrophages. J Exp Med 171: 35–47

Spertini F, Spits H, Geha RS (1991) Staphylococcal exotoxins deliver activation signals to human T-cell clones via major histocompatibility complex class II molecules. Proc Natl Acad Sci USA 88 (in press)

Todd J, Fishaut M, Kapral F, Welch T (1978) Toxic-shock syndrome associated with phage-group 1 staphylococci. Lancet 2: 1116–1118

Tracey JT, Fong Y, Hesse DG, Manogue KR, Lee AT, Kuo GC, Lowry SF, Cerami A (1987) Anti cachectin/TNF monoclonal antibodies prevent septic shock during lethal bacteraemia. Nature 330: 662–664

Tracey KJ, Beutler B, Lowry SF, Merryweather J, Wolpe S, Milsark IW, Hairi IJ, Fahey TJ, Zentella A, Albert JD, Cerami A (1986) Shock and tissue injury induced by recombinant human cachectin. Science 234: 470–473

Trede N, Geha RS, Chatila T (1991) Transcriptional activation of monokine genes by MHC class II ligands. J Immunol 146: 2310–2315

Uchiyama T, Kamagata Y, Wakai M, Yoshioka M, Fujikawa H, Igarashi H (1986) Study of the biological activities of toxic shock syndrome toxin-1. I. Proliferative response and interleukin-2 production by T cells stimulated with the toxin. Microbiol Immunol 30: 469–483

Uchiyama T, Imanishi K, Saito S, Arrake M, Yan X-J, Fujikawa H, Igarashi H, Kato H, Obata F, Kashiwagi N, Inoko H (1989a) Activation of human T cells by toxic shock syndrome toxin-1: the toxin-binding structures expressed on human lymphoid cells acting as accessory cells are HLA class II molecules. Eur J Immunol 19: 1803–1809

Uchiyama T, Tadakuma T, Imanishi K, Araake M, Saito S, Yan X-J, Fujikawa H, Igarashi H, Yamaura N (1989b) Activation of murine T cells by toxic shock syndrome toxin-1. The toxin-binding structure expressed on murine accessory cells are MHC class II molecules. J Immunol 143: 3175–3182

Ullrich A, Schlessinger J (1990) Signal transduction by receptors with tyrosine kinase activity. Cell 61: 203–212

Staphylococcal Enterotoxin-Dependent Cell-Mediated Cytotoxicity

T. Kalland[1,2], G. Hedlund[1,2], M. Dohlsten[1,2], and P. A. Lando[1]

1 Introduction

The relationship between microorganisms and mammals is regulated by a complex interplay between pathogenic and protective mechanisms. The primary defense against bacteria is mainly constituted of mechanical barriers, such as intact epithelial membranes, and nonspecific immune mechanisms, for example granulocytes and macrophages. Bacteria generally cause disease when these barriers are overridden. It has recently become increasingly clear, however, that specific immune responses mediated by antigen-specific T and B lymphocytes are of critical importance as a physiological barrier capable of controlling the growth of invading bacteria. Patients with selective defects in specific immunity suffer from an increased susceptibility to bacteria, including those that are non-pathogenic in the normal host. Insight into the strategies employed by bacteria to evade immune recognition is accumulating. Several bacterial exoproteins have been reported to induce polyclonal activation of T or B lymphocytes with subsequent incapability to mount a specific immune response (Alouf 1986;

[1] Kabi Pharmacia Therapeutics AB, Scheelevägen 22, 22363 Lund, Sweden
[2] Department of Tumor Immunology, The Wallenberg Laboratory, University of Lund, 22363 Lund, Sweden

REIMANN et al. 1990). Moreover, excessive lymphokine production results in harmful effects on the integrity of tissues facilitating penetration of bacteria. Of particular interest is the description of bacterial products which interact with key elements of the specific immune system such as antibodies, MHC antigens, or T cell receptors. Staphylococcal and streptococcal cell wall proteins A and G have been shown to bind in a specific manner to immunoglobulins, and *Branhamella catarrhalis* and *Haemophilus influenza* interact with IgD on the surface of B lymphocytes (BOYLE 1990). Recently, staphylococcal enterotoxins (SEs) and some related proteins have been shown to utilize MHC class II antigens as receptors on mammalian cells (FISCHER et al. 1989; FRASER 1989; MOLLICK et al. 1989). The complexes, made up of toxin and MHC protein stimulate large numbers of T cells (WHITE et al. 1989), and the subsequent excessive production of lymphokines may at least partly be responsible for their toxicity (MARRACK et al. 1990). In the following we will describe a more subtle result of this interaction, the staphylococcal enterotoxin-dependent cellular cytotoxicity (SDCC) reaction, a possible mechanism for certain bacteria to evade specific immune recognition.

2 SDCC: A Cytotoxic Mechanism Induced by Bacterial Exoproteins

The potent T cell activating properties of SEs have been known for 20 years (PEARY et al. 1970) and the molecular requirements for and consequences of this activation are currently being characterized in great detail, as reviewed elsewhere in this volume. SEA induces a variety of functions associated with T cell activity, notably the production of lymphokines such as interleukin-2 (IL-2), interferon-γ (IFN-γ) and tumor necrosis factor (TNF) (CARLSSON and SJÖGREN 1985; FISCHER et al. 1990). In common with many T cell mitogens, SEA also induces the lytic function of cytotoxic T cells (ZEHAVI-WILLNER and BERKE 1986; FLEISCHER and SCHREZENMEIER 1988). During studies of activation requirements of antigen-specific cytotoxic T cells, we observed that inclusion of SEA in the cytotoxicity assay altered their apparent target cell specificity (DOHLSTEN et al. 1990). Human allospecific T cell lines, which under normal conditions showed strict specificity for HLA-A2, demonstrated strong cytotoxicity against the irrelevant HLA-A2$^-$ HLA-A3$^+$ DR$^+$ Raji target cell and increased cytotoxicity superimposed on that against the specific HLA-A2$^+$ DR$^+$ BSM target cell in the presence of SEA (Fig. 1). The SDCC effect was consistently observed at concentrations as low as $10^{-13} M$ SEA and maximal effects were reached at about $5 \times 10^{-12} M$ (Fig. 1). It was likely that a large fraction of T cells was recruited as effector cells in the reaction since significant cytotoxicity was observed at effector-target ratios below 5:1. This was further strengthened by the fact that the SDCC was a rapid phenomenon. Detectable lysis of target cells was seen after less than 30 min and half-maximal and plateau levels were essentially reached within 1 and 2 h, respectively (HEDLUND et al. 1990).

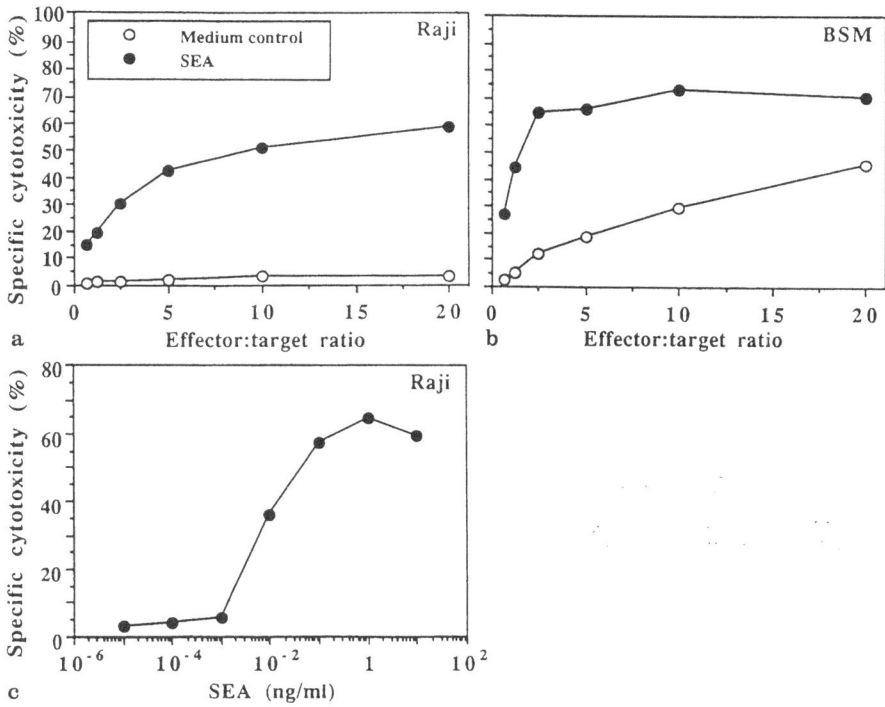

Fig. 1 a–c. a, b SEA-dependent cell-mediated cytotoxicity by a HLA-A2-specific human T cell line against Raji (HLA-A2⁻) and BSM (HLA-A2⁺) target cells in the presence (●) or absence (○) of SEA (1 ng/ml). **c** Cytotoxicity at effector: target ratio 10:1 against Raji cells in the presence of varying concentrations of SEA

3 Effector Cells Mediating SDCC

Characterization of SDCC effector cell phenotype by analysis of T and natural killer (NK) cell clones revealed that the response was mediated exclusively by T cells (DOHLSTEN et al. 1990). None of a number of NK cell clones could be activated by SEA or mediate SDCC in the presence of any member of the SE family (LANDO et al. 1990; DOHLSTEN et al. 1990). The lack of SDCC activity in these NK clones does not exclude the participation of subpopulations of NK cells not growing under the cloning conditions we have used. However it is rather unlikely that NK cells mediate SDCC since NK cells purified by cell sorting from peripheral blood lymphocytes (PBL) did not show any sign of SDCC activity (LANDO et al. 1991). NK cells were activated to exert lymphocyte-activated killer (LAK)-like cytotoxic activity in 3–5 day cultures of PBL stimulated with SEA, but NK cells isolated from such cultures did not mediate SDCC (LANDO et al. 1991).

Analysis of CD4$^+$ or CD8$^+$ cells and use of cloned T cells clearly indicated that both the major populations of T cells were able to mediate SDCC (DOHLSTEN et al. 1990; HEDLUND et al. 1990). Whether this is a reflection of a facilitated interaction between the CD4 effector cells and MHC class II on the target cells has not been directly addressed. The SDCC phenomenon was not restricted to SEA but could be induced by all SEs examined. Since the response to SEs has been shown to be clonally variable (FLEISCHER and SCHREZENMEIER 1988; WHITE et al. 1989; LANDO et al. 1990), we used activation with different SEs as a tool to generate T cell lines and clones with selective reactivity towards SEs. When examined in the SDCC assay, some of these cell lines and clones showed strict reactivity with a certain SE with virtually no cross-reactivity with others. It has been convincingly shown that SEs activate T cells to proliferation and lymphokine production through interaction with variable segments of the T cell receptor β chain. The data summarized above strongly indicate that a similar interaction also activates T cells effective in SDCC.

4 Target Structure in SDCC

The ability of SEs to direct T cells of irrelevant nominal specificity towards certain target cells correlated with expression of the HLA-DR molecule, which was the major MHC class II-encoded protein expressed on the cell lines used as targets. Blocking studies with monoclonal antibodies (mAbs) directed to different cell surface structures demonstrated that the mAb G8, which has been shown to interact with a SEA binding site on the HLA-DR molecule (FISCHER et al. 1989), strongly inhibited SDCC (Table 1). In contrast, the HB96 mAb, which interacts with a monomorphic MHC class II determinant unrelated to the SEA binding epitope (FISCHER et al. 1989), and mAbs towards MHC class I or CD23 did not show any inhibitory activity. The MHC class II-negative mutant of Raji RJ 2.2.5 was completely resistant to SDCC, while the parental Raji cell line was an excellent target. Furthermore, L cells transfected with DR2A or DR2B, but not mock-transfected L cells, were sensitive to SDCC. CD4 and CD8 T cells were equally effective in killing DR2 transfected L cells. Since human CD8 molecules do not interact with murine MHC class I (SAMBERG et al. 1989), the CD8 molecule was apparently not of significant importance for the SDCC effector function. MHC class II antigens are the only receptors for SEs on mammalian cells described so far (FISCHER et al. 1989; MOLLICK et al. 1989; FRASER 1989). The data reported here demonstrate that MHC class II antigens are necessary and sufficient target structures for the SDCC phenomenon. However, we have recently demonstrated that colon carcinoma cell lines which lack MHC class II antigens detectable by flow cytometry, immunoprecipitation, or northern blotting may be targets in SDCC in the presence of SEB (DOHLSTEN et al. 1991b). It is possible that the acute enterotoxic effects of SEs are mediated through this

Table 1. HLA-DR is a target molecule in SDCC

	Target	Additive		Cytotoxicity		
		SEA	mAb	A(%)	B(%)	C(%)
Experiment 1	Raji	—	—	1	0	0
	Raji	+	—	30	19	14
	Raji	+	HB96	31	23	16
	Raji	+	G8	8	6	3
	Raji	+	W6/32	37	28	19
	Raji	+	CD23	40	27	19
Experiment 2	Raji	—	—	2	0	0
	Raji	+	—	43	30	22
	RJ2.2.5	—	—	10	11	8
	RJ2.2.5	+	—	12	9	6
Experiment 3	LDR2A	—	—	0	0	0
	LDR2A	+	—	24	18	8
	LDR2B	—	—	0	0	0
	LDR2B	+	—	25	18	4
	L cells	—	—	0	0	0
	L cells	+	—	0	0	0

Cytotoxicity of an anti-HLA-A2-specific T cell line against the indicated target cells. The different mAb were added in the cytotoxicity assay at saturating dilutions and SEA was added in the assay at a concentration of 0.1 ng/ml (Exp. 1), 1 ng/ml (Exp. 2) or 100 ng/ml (Exp. 3). The E:T ratios A, B and C were 20:1, 10:1, and 5:1 in Exps. 1 and 2, 30:1, 10:1, and 3:1 in Exp. 3

putative novel SE receptor. By chemical modification of SEB, Fleischer and coworkers have shown that the enterotoxic effect of SEB can be dissociated from its T cell mitogenic properties (ALBER et al. 1990).

5 Accessory Molecules Participating in SDCC

Efficient antigen-specific recognition by T cells requires, in addition to the T cell receptor (TCR), a number of accessory moelcules. It is generally believed that the adhesion molecules increase the avidity of the interaction between the TCR and the MHC-antigen complex and may provide costimulatory signals (SPRINGER 1990). Most interesting, the binding of toxic shock syndrome toxin-1 (TSST-1) to MHC class II was reported to enhance the interaction between the CD11a/CD18 and ICAM-1 (CD54) adhesion molecules. The involvement of the MHC class II antigens and the TCR indicate that the activation processes of SEs and antigen peptides are closely related. Recent studies have indicated, however, that the interaction sites of SEs with the MHC class II antigens and the TCR are different from those interacting with peptides during conventional MHC-restricted T cell recognition of protein antigens (DELLABONA et al. 1990; CHOI et al. 1990). To

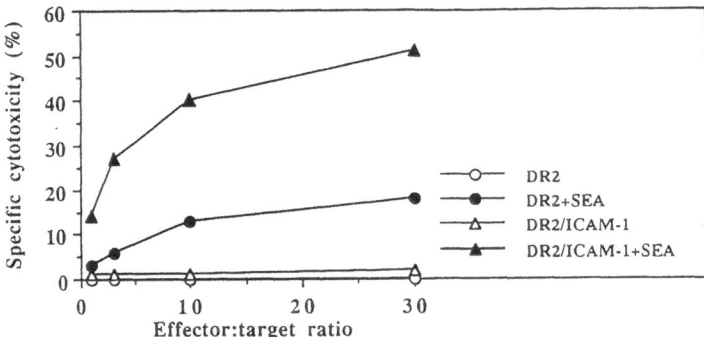

Fig. 2. SEA-dependent cell-mediated cytotoxicity of a human SEA responding T cell line against L cells transfected with HLA-DR2 or HLA-DR2 and ICAM-1 preincubated (*filled symbols*) or not (*open symbols*) with 100 ng/ml SEA

examine the importance of the adhesion molecules ICAM-1 and LFA-3 (CD58), we used double transfected L cells expressing both HLA-DR molecules and an adhesion molecules as target cells in SDCC (DOHLSTEN et al. 1991a). Human SEA-selective T cell lines demonstrated a low but significant cytotoxicity against SEA-coated HLA-DR transfected L cells. However, when L cells were cotransfected with ICAM-1, they served as excellent targets in SDCC, being killed at an effector-target ratio 30 times lower than the single DR transfectant. (Fig. 2). Dose response analysis demonstrated that a 1000-fold lower concentration of SEA was sufficient to obtain equivalent levels of lysis in the double vs the single transfected target cells. Similar results were obtained with L cells transfected with other DR alleles. The insensitivity of single transfected target cells could not be overcome by increasing the concentration of SEA. The strong cytolysis of the DR2/ICAM-1 L cells could be inhibited by addition of mAbs directed towards the ICAM-1, CD11a, or CD18 antigens but not by mAbs towards MHC class I, CD2, CD11b, or CD11c, indicating that the CD11a/CD18 was the major receptor for ICAM-1 on the target cells used. This suggested that efficient targeting of CTL requires coexpression of MHC class II antigens and ICAM-1. In a similar analysis of the role of LFA-3, utilizing CHO cells transfected with HLA-DR and LFA-3 genes, analogous findings were obtained (GJÖRLOFF et al., manuscript in preparation. However, while the dependence of ICAM-1 on L cells was the same for CD4$^+$ and CD8$^+$ cells, CD4$^+$ cells were more dependent on LFA-3 for efficient lysis of CHO cells. A reasonable interpretation would be that these accessory molecules can alternate in provision of the necessary secondary stabilization of the interaction mediated by SEA. Depending on the availability of the receptor or ligand on target and effector cells, ICAM-1 or LFA-3 can be preferentially utilized. Moreover, it is likely that even other adhesion molecules are able to participate in the SDCC reaction. Several lymphokines participate in the regulation of the surface expression of adhesion molecules, including IFN-γ and TNF. Activation of T lymphocytes with SEA induces the production of IFN-γ and TNF-α (CARLSSON and SJÖGREN 1985; FISCHER et al. 1989) which may result in enhanced surface expression of both MHC class II antigens, ICAM-1, and LFA-3 on the target cell. This may recruit additional target cells wich would otherwise escape destruction by SDCC.

6 Freshly Isolated Tumor Cells and Normal Cells as Targets in SDCC

A variety of tumor cells have been examined as targets in the SDCC reaction. Lymphoblastoid cells lines served as excellent targets, most likely dependent on their high expression of both MHC class II antigens and adhesion molecules. Moreover, freshly isolated leukemia cells and MHC class II-expressing renal and colorectal carcinomas have successfully been used as SDCC targets (HEDLUND et al. 1990; LANDO et al. unpublished observation). This finding makes it terapting to speculate if SEs can be used for specific elimination of tumor cells expressing MHC class II. In particular, SDCC might be utilized in conjunction with IFN or TNF which are able to induce MHC class II and adhesion molecule expression in tumor cells (MORTARINI et al. 1990). The side effects associated with administration of SEs are probably at least partly the consequence of T cell activation

Table 2. Monocytes, B lymphocytes, and activated T lymphocytes are targets in SDCC

	Target	% DR[a]	SEA[b]	Cytotoxicity at E:T ratio (%)		
				10	5	2.5
Experiment 1	Raji	100	—	0	0	0
	Raji		+	65	50	26
	T_{act}	62	—	0	0	0
	T_{act}		+	29	18	15
	Monocytes	86	—	0	1	1
	Monocytes		+	46	38	26
Experiment 2	Raji	100	—	2	1	2
	Raji		+	60	49	32
	T	4	—	0	0	0
	T		+	0	0	0
	T_{act}	38	—	0	0	0
	T_{act}		+	32	33	26
	B	100	—	10	10	2
	B		+	72	47	41

The effector cells were a SEA-selective T cell line
[a] Relative frequency of HLA-DR$^+$ among target cells as determined by flow cytometry
[b] Target cells were preincubated with (+) or without SEA (−) (100 ng/ml)

(MARRACK et al. 1990), and systemic effects might be ameliorated by targeted delivery of SEs to the tumor.

To investigate whether SDCC would be potentially destructive even to normal cells, we analyzed the SDCC capacity of SEA- selective T cell lines against autologous monocytes, B cells, and activated MHC class II-expressing T cells. It was found that these cells were sensitive to SDCC when preincubated with SEs (Table 2). In contrast, resting T cells, which do not express detectable amounts of MHC class II antigens, were not lysed in the presence of SEA.

7 Induction of SDCC In Vivo

While the T cell activating properties of SEs have been extensively studied in vitro, rather limited information is available concerning the effects on the immune system in vivo. To explore the SDCC phenomenon in vivo, C57B1/6 mice were injected i.v. with varying doses of SEA, and the cytotoxic activity of spleen lymphocytes against I-A- and I-E-expressing mouse tumor cells was examined at different time intervals. Lymphocytes from mice injected with 10 µg SEA showed

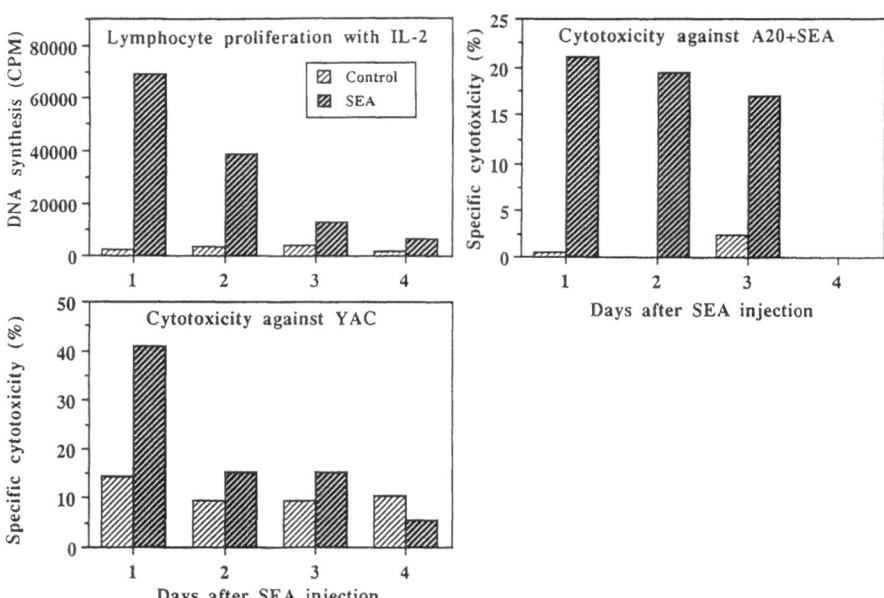

Fig. 3. Lymphocyte activation in vivo with SEA. C57B1/6 mice were injected i.v. with 10 µg SEA and spleen lymphocytes examined ex vivo for proliferative response to exogenous IL-2 (20 U/ml) and cytotoxicity against A20 cells preincubated with SEA (10 µg/ml) or YAC-1 cells. Effector: target ratio 100:1

negligible cytotoxic activity against the relatively NK-resistant lymphoma A20. However, when A20 cells were preincubated with SEA, they served as excellent targets, indicating that SDCC effector cells were induced in vivo (Fig. 3). SDCC activity was prominent at 24 h after injection, the earliest time tested. High activity was retained for about 3 days and declined on day 4 after a single injection. No SDCC activity was detected in mice injected with excipient control. Evidence of enhanced NK activity, as detected by cytotoxic acitivity towards the NK target YAC-1, was seen at day 1 but decreased to control levels at day 2. The mechanism behind the enhanced NK activity was not studied, but was most likely the result of activation secondary to IL-2 produced by SEA-activated T cells. In vitro activation of human NK cells required the presence of T cells (LANDO et al. 1991). Moreover, we have previously shown that SEA activation of mouse NK cells in vitro was blocked by antibodies towards the IL-2 receptor (BHILADVALA et al. 1991). Recent studies have documented that injection of SEB into neonatal or adult mice may result in immunosuppression, either generalized due to poly-clonal T cell activation or specific due to clonal deletion or anergization of T cells expressing TCR-V_β chains reacting with SEB (DONELLY and ROGERS 1982; WHITE et al. 1989; MARRACK et al. 1990; RELLAHAN et al. 1990). In the latter case, SEB-reactive lymphocytes were not able to respond to exogenously provided IL-2 although IL-2 receptor expression was apparently normal. In contrast, we obser-ved strong proliferative responses to IL-2 after priming the mice with SEA (Fig. 3). Several differences between the experimental settings existed, and it may be interesting to define the parameters of SE administration that lead alternatively to T cell activation or the induction of tolerance.

8 Biological Interpretation of SDCC: A Mechanism for Bacteria to Evade Specific Immune Recognition

The highly conserved interaction of SEs with two of the major players of the immune system is remarkable in light of the polymorphism of these structures. Clearly the bacteria must derive some advantage from the production of toxins of this type (MARRACK and KAPPLER 1990). The immune system is not only confronted with pathogens present extracellularly (bacteria, fungi, parasites), but also with intracellularly harbored viruses and prokaryotes. The MHC class I and II molecules have evolved to serve as systems which allow separate pathways for antigen processing of intracellularly and extracellularly derived proteins and selective presentation of these to CD8 cytotoxic and CD4 T helper cells, respectively (KOURILSKY and CLAVERIE 1989). Not surprisingly, pathogens have developed strategies intended to circumvent these defense mechanisms. Among several mechanisms utilized by viruses to perturb efficient immune recognition, we find one of particular interest for the present discussion. Adenovirus down-regulates surface expression of MHC class I in infected host cells by its E19

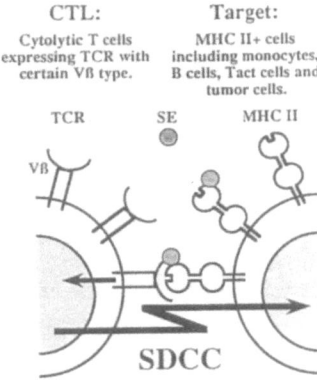

CTL: Target:

Cytolytic T cells   MHC II+ cells
expressing TCR with   including monocytes,
certain Vß type.   B cells, Tact cells and
                          tumor cells.

TCR   SE   MHC II

Vß

SDCC

Fig. 4. General outline of the SDCC reaction. SDCC requires initial binding of SEs to MHC class II molecules and subsequent interaction with T cells expressing particular TCR V_β families. The SDCC phenomenon results in rapid killing at the SE presenting target cell

protein, which retains MHC class I molecules in the endoplasmatic reticulum. The virus thereby prevents effective presentation of viral peptides to T lymphocytes (MARTENS et al. 1989). MHC class II antigens are pivotal for presentation of peptides derived from extracellular sources such as bacteria. The binding of SEs to conserved regions of MHC class II antigens and activation of SDCC with subsequent elimination of the cells capable of presenting bacterial antigens is an additional example of the logic created by the evolutionary interplay between the immune system and the environment. While polyclonal activation of T cells and profound lymphokine production definitely may pertubate an immune response, the SDCC response, which results in the specific destruction of MHC class II-expressing antigen presenting cells, appears as a more distinct way of avoiding recognition by T cells. The relative contribution of these mechanisms to the host-bacterial interaction is presently unknown. Although we have shown that the SDCC phenomenon is detectable in vivo in response to SEs, its relevance awaits studies in infectious models in vivo. Presently, it can only be speculated if the lessons learned from studies of the immunological properties of SEs can be taken advantage of for therapeutic purposes. In particular, if local delivery of SEs can be achieved, they may be useful for down-regulation of autoimmune processes and perhaps also for activation of tumor infiltrating lymphocytes in situ.

References

Alber G, Hammer DK, Fleischer B (1990) Relationship between enterotoxic- and T-lymphocyte-stimulating activity of staphylococcal enterotoxin B. J Immunol 144: 4501–4506

Alouf JE (1986) Interaction of bacterial protein toxins with host defence mechanisms. In: Bacterial protein toxins. Falmagne P, Alouf JE, Fehrenbach FJ, Jeljaszewicz J (eds) Fischer, Stuttgart, pp 121–130

Bhiladvala P, Belfrage H, Petersson C, Hedlund G, Dohlsten M, Kalland T (1991) Selective activation of T cell derived LAK cells by staphylococcal enterotoxin A. Manuscript in preparation

Boyle MDP (1990) Bacterial immunoglobulin-binding proteins. Academic Press, San Diego

Carlsson R, Sjögren HO (1985) Kinetics of IL-2 and interferon-γ production, expression of IL-2 receptors and cell proliferation in human mononuclear cells exposed to staphylococcal enterotoxin A. Cell Immunol 96: 175–182

Choi Y, Herman A, Diguisto D, Wade T, Marrack P, Kappler J (1990) Residues of the variable region of the T cell receptor β-chain that interact with S aureus toxin superantigens. Nature 346: 471–473

Dellabona P, Peccoud J, Kappler J, Marrack P, Benoist C, Mathis D (1990) Superantigens interact with MHC class II molecules outside of the antigen groove. Cell 62: 1115–1121

Dohlsten M, Lando PA, Hedlund G, Trowsdale J, Kalland T (1990) Targeting of human cytotoxic T lymphocytes to MHC class II expressing cells by staphylococcal enterotoxins. Immunology 71: 96–100

Dohlsten M, Hedlund G, Lando PA, Trowsdale J, Altman D, Patarroya M, Fischer H, Kalland T (1991a) Role of the adhesion molecule ICAM-1 (CD54) in staphylococcal enterotoxin-mediated cytotoxicity. Eur J Immunol 21: 131–135

Dohlsten M, Hedlund G, Segren S, Lando PA, Herrman T, Kelly AP, Kalland T (1991b) Human MHC Class II⁻ colon carcinoma cells presents staphylococcal superantigens to cytotoxic T lymphocytes: evidence for a novel enterotoxic receptor. Eur J Immunol 21: 1229–1233

Donelly RP, Rogers TJ (1982) Immune suppression induced by staphylococcal enterotoxin B. Cell Immunol 72: 166–173

Fischer H, Dohlsten M, Lindvall M, Sjögren HO, Carlsson R (1989) Binding of staphylococcal enterotoxin A to HLA-DR on B cell lines. J Immunol 142: 3151–3155

Fischer H, Dohlsten M, Andersson U, Hedlund G, Ericsson PO, Hansson J, Sjögren HO (1990) Production of TNF-α and TNF-β by staphylococcal enterotoxin A activated human T cells. J Immunol 144: 4663–4666

Fleischer B, Schrezenmeier H (1988) T cell stimulation by staphylococcal enterotoxins. J Exp Med 167: 1697–1707

Fraser JD (1989) High affinity binding of staphylococcal enterotoxins A and B to HLA-DR. Nature 339: 221–224

Hedlund G, Dohlsten M, Lando PA, Kalland T (1990) Staphylococcal enterotoxins direct and trigger CTL killing of autologous HLA-DR⁺ mononuclear leukocytes and freshly prepared leukemia cells. Cell Immunol 129: 426–434

Kourilsky P, Claverie JM (1989) MHC-antigen interaction: what does the T cell receptor see? Adv Immunol 45: 107–194

Lando PA, Dohlsten M, Kalland T, Sjögren HO, Carlsson R (1990) The TCR- CD3 complex is required for activation of human lymphocytes with staphylococcal enterotoxin A. Scand J Immunol 31: 133–138

Lando PA, Hedlund G, Dohlsten M, Kalland T (1991) Bacterial superantigens as anti-tumor agents: induction of tumor cytotoxicity in human lymphocytes by staphylococcal enterotoxin A. Cancer Immunol Immunother 33: 231–237

Marrack P, Kappler J (1990) The staphylococcal enterotoxins and their relatives. Science 248: 704–711

Marrack P, Blackman M, Kushmir E, Kappler J (1990) The toxicity of staphylococcal enterotoxin B in mice is mediated by T cells. J Exp Med 171: 455–464

Martens I, Nilsson T, Petersson PA (1989) Adenovirus proteins and MHC expression. Adv Cancer Res 52: 151–163

Mollick JA, Cook RG, Rich RR (1989) Class II MHC molecules are specific receptors for staphylococcus enterotoxin A. Science 244: 817–821

Mortarini R, Belli F, Parmiani G, Anichini A (1990) Cytokine-mediated modulation of HLA-class II, ICAM-1, LFA-3 and tumor-associated antigen profile of melanoma cell. Comparison with antiproliferative activity by rIL-1β, rTNF-α, rIL-4 and their combinations. Int J Cancer 45: 334–341

Peary DL, Adler WH, Smith RT (1970) The mitogenic effect of endotoxin and staphylococcal enterotoxin B on mouse spleen cells and human peripheral blood lymphocytes. J Immunol 105: 1453–1457

Reimann J, Claesson MH, Qvirin N (1990) Suppression of the immune response by microorganisms. Scand J Immunol 31: 543–546

Rellahan BL, Jones LA, Kruisbeek AM, Fry AM, Matis LA (1990) In vivo induction of anergy in peripheral Vβ8⁺ T cells by staphylococcal enterotoxin B. J Exp Med 172: 1091–1100

Samberg N, Scarlett EC, Stauss H (1989) The α3 domain of MHC class I molecules plays a critical role in cytotoxic T lymphocyte stimulation. Eur J Immunol 19: 2349–2354

Springer T (1990) Adhesion receptors of the immune system. Nature 346: 425–434

White J, Herman A, Pullen AM, Kubo R, Kappler JW, Marrack P (1989) The V_β specific superantigen staphylococcal enterotoxin B: stimulation of mature T cells and clonal deletion in neonatal mice Cell 56: 27–35

Zehavi-Willner T, Berke G (1986) The mitogenic activity of staphylococcal enterotoxin B (SEB): a monovalent T cell mitogen that stimulates cytolytic T lymphocytes but cannot mediate their lytic interaction. J Immunol 137: 2682–2687

CD4/CD8 Coreceptor-Independent Costimulator-Dependent Triggering of SEB-Reactive Murine T Cells*

K. Heeg, T. Miethke, P. Bader, S. Bendigs, C. Wahl, and H. Wagner

1 Introduction

Conventional antigen binds as a processed peptide fragment in the groove of the responder allele of the major histocompatibility complex (MHC) molecule and is recognized by the variable regions of T cell receptors (TCRs) of clonally distributed T lymphocytes (Bjorkman et al. 1987; Buus et al. 1987; Townsend et al. 1986; Davis and Bjorkman 1988; Matis 1990). An array of coreceptors (CD4, CD8, LFA-1, CD2, etc.) further strengthens the association between TCR and MHC-bound peptide antigen and provides additional signals necessary for T cell activation and triggering of T cell function (Bierer et al. 1989; Veillette et al. 1989; Staunton et al. 1989; Meuer et al. 1984b). A second category of TCR-unlinked costimulatory signals generated by antigen-presenting cells (APC) critically controls primary T cell activation (Bretscher and Cohn 1970; Geppert et al. 1990). Occupancy of the TCR and coreceptors without an APC-derived costimulus anergizes rather than activates antigen-reactive resting T cells (Jenkins et al. 1988; Schwartz 1989; Gaspari et al. 1988).

Institute of Medical Microbiology and Hygiene, Technical University of Munich, Trogerstraße 4a, 8000 Munich 80, FRG
* This work was supported by the Sonderforschungsbereich (SFB)322 of the Deutsche Forschungsgemeinschaft

Superantigens such as staphylococcal enterotoxin B (SEB) essentially bypass the conventional antigen presentation route (MARRACK and KAPPLER 1990). Rather, they behave like bifunctional agents: using a conserved binding region they associate as unprocessed protein with class II MHC molecules (FLEISCHER and SCHREZENMEIER 1988; FRASER 1989; MOLLICK et al. 1989; FLEISCHER et al. 1989; RUSSELL et al. 1990; HERRMANN et al. 1989; SCHOLL et al. 1989a, b, 1990; KARP et al. 1990; FISCHER et al. 1989). Enterotoxins bound to MHC class II molecules then specifically interact with certain V_β-encoded domains of the TCR (CHOI et al. 1990; YAGI et al. 1990; JANEWAY et al. 1989; KAPPLER et al. 1989). Although superantigen binding to class II MHC antigens can be readily detected, association of soluble enterotoxins to TCR is not brought about, thus suggesting binding of a low-affinity soluble enterotoxin with the TCR. This novel mode of antigen presentation prompted us to investigate the requirements of CD4/CD8 coreceptors and of TCR-independent costimulator activities during SEB-mediated T lymphocyte activation, their role in thymic selection processes, and triggering of lytic effector function.

2 Coreceptor Requirements During SEB-Induced Primary T Cell Activation

In conventional T cell activation, the class of the presenting MHC molecule dictates the CD4/CD8 phenotype of the responding T cell (SWAIN 1983). Only a minority of CD8 or CD4 T cells ($< 5\%$) is activated by class II or class I MHC alloantigens, respectively (SPRENT et al. 1986; MIZUOCHI et al. 1986; HEEG et al. 1987). If this rule holds for superantigens, preferentially CD4 T cells ought to be activated by MHC class II-bound SEB. However, it was recognized that CD8 T lymphocytes could be activated equally well as CD4 cells by SEB on syngeneic feeder cells (FLEISCHER and SCHREZENMEIER 1988; HERRMANN et al. 1990). Figure 1 depicts an experiment of this type, in which cell sorter-purified CD8 T cells were activated by SEB. Note that SEB-induced activation of CD8 lymphocytes could not be blocked with monoclonal anti-CD8 antibodies which readily abrogate the activation of CD8 T cells stimulated with class I MHC alloantigens or class I MHC-restricted antigens (MACDONALD et al. 1981; HERRMANN et al. 1990) (Fig. 1). On the contrary, these monoclonal antibodies (mAb) enhanced dose-dependently the proliferative response of CD8 T cells (Fig. 1). To exclude the possibility that only a minor subset of CD8 T cells responds to SEB, we used the limiting dilution approach to measure the number of SEB inducible CD4 and CD8 T cells. The results shown in Table 1 reveal that 15% of anti-CD3 inducible CD8 T cells gave rise to proliferating progeny after stimulation with SEB; this number was further enhanced in the $V_\beta 8$-expressing CD8 T lymphocyte pool (Table 1). Thus, SEB bound to class II MHC antigens effectively stimulates resting CD8 T cells bearing the appropriate V_β-encoded TCR. Since anti-CD8 mAb do not block this

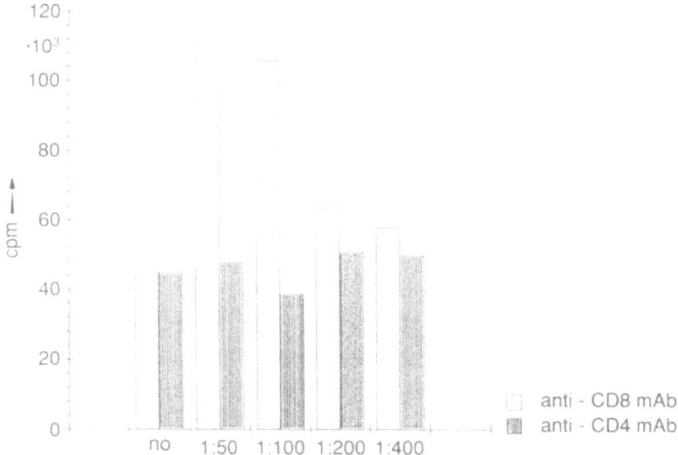

Fig. 1. Coreceptor-independent activation of SEB-reactive CD8$^+$ T cells. A population of 5000 cell sorter purified CD8 T lymphocytes from B6 mice were incubated with syngeneic feeder cells and SEB in the presence of a serial dilution of affinity-purified anti-CD8 (*open columns*) or anti-CD4 (*solid columns*) mAb. After 5 days the cultures were pulsed with [^{3}H] thymidine. The mean cpm values of six replicate cultures are given

Table 1. Frequency analysis of SEB inducible CD4 and CD8 T lymphocytes

Responder T cell	Stimulation	1/Frequency of proliferating T cells
CD4$^+$	Anti-CD3 hybridoma	7.2
CD4$^+$	SEB	100.2
CD4$^+$F23$^+$	Anti-CD3 hybridoma	3.8
CD4$^+$F23$^+$	SEB	12.9
CD8$^+$	Anti-CD3 hybridoma	1.4
CD8$^+$	SEB	10.0
CD8$^+$F23$^+$	Anti-CD3 hybridoma	2.4
CD8$^+$F23$^+$	SEB	6.0

Cell sorter-purified CD4 or CD8 T cells were stimulated under limiting dilution conditions with 5000 irradiated anti-CD3 mAb producing hybridoma cells or 10 µg/ml SEB in the presence of irradiated syngeneic feeder cells. After 7 days the microcultures were pulsed with [^{3}H] thymidine and the proliferative response was recorded. From the fraction of negative cultures the frequency was calculated

activation, it follows that SEB recognition by resting CD8 T cells is CD8 coreceptor-independent.

3 Costimulator Requirements During Primary Activation of CD8 T Lymphocytes with SEB

Studies with mAb fragments revealed that engagement of the TCR without cross-linking is insufficient for T cell triggering (KAYE et al. 1983; MEUER et al. 1984a). Accordingly, incubation of resting CD8 T cells with soluble SEB, which posseses only a monovalent binding site for the TCR, in the absence of feeder cells does not result in T cell triggering (Table 2). To construct a matrix of SEB capable of cross-linking TCRs, we covalently bound SEB to CNBr-activated sepharose beads. While both soluble SEB in the presence of syngeneic feeder cells and sepharose-linked anti-CD3 mAb triggered CD8 T cells to proliferation with high efficiency (MIETHKE et al. 1991), a proliferative response of resting CD8 T cells incubated with SEB immobilized on sepharose was only recorded at high ($> 10^4$) cell densities (Fig. 2). In addition, this response was blocked by mAb specific for MHC class II molecules (data not given), suggesting that contaminating class II-positive cells are critically involved in the response to immobilized SEB. At first glance these results suggest that the binding affinity of immobilized SEB to the TCR does not exceed the threshold necessary for triggering resting T cells. Weak TCR-linked signals delivered via anti-CD3 or anti-α/β TCR mAb become substantially enhanced by coengagement of the CD8 coreceptor via immobilized anti-CD8 mAb (EICHMANN et al. 1987; MIETHKE and KOSSIK, personal communication). We therefore tested whether co-coupling of anti-CD8 mAb together with SEB to sepharose beads would provide such a synergistic effect. Although sepharose-immobilized anti-CD8 mAb clearly enhanced responses induced by suboptimal concentrations of immobilized anti-α/β mAb (data not given), such an effect was not seen with SEB (Fig. 3a). Thus, SEB immobilized on sepharose beads fails to activate resting CD8 T cells even if the coreceptor (CD8)

Table 2. Soluble SEB without feeder cells fails to trigger resting CD8 T cells

Responder cells	Feeder cells	Proliferative response (cpm)
CD8$^+$ T cells	—	769
CD8$^+$ T cells	+	91 092

Resting CD8$^+$ T cells (1000/well) were activated by SEB (10 µg/ml) in the presence or absence of irradiated syngeneic feeder cells (5 × 10^4/well). The cultures were pulsed with [^{3}H] thymidine during the last 8 h of a 7 day culture period

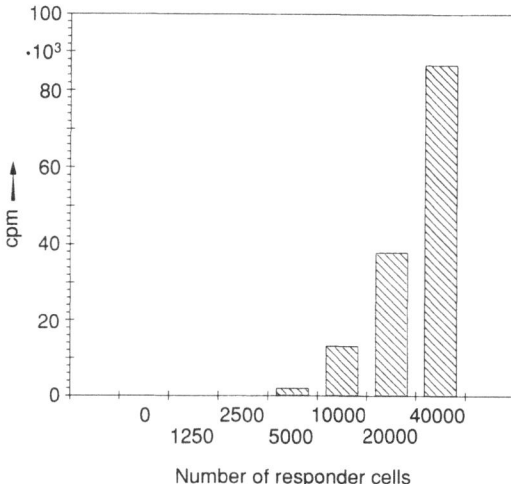

Fig. 2. Immobilized SEB fails to activate resting CD8 T cells. Graded numbers of cell sorter-purified $CD8^+$ T cells were activated with sepharose beads (0.25 mg/ml) coupled with SEB (2.5 mg SEB/10 mg sepharose beads), cultured for 7 days, and pulsed with [^{3}H] thymidine for 8 h

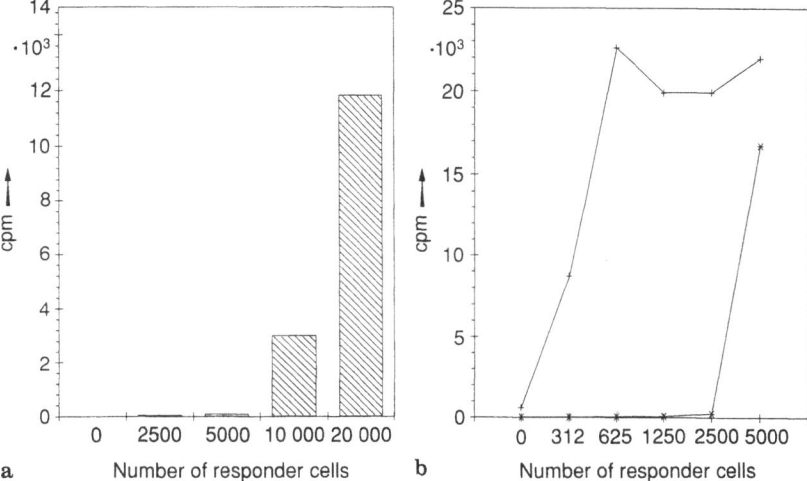

Fig. 3 a, b. Cross-linking of coreceptors does not restore induction of proliferation in CD8 T cells triggered by immobilized SEB. **a** Resting cell sorter-purified $CD8^+$ T cells were cultured for 7 days in titrated numbers and activated with sepharose beads (0.25 mg/ml) coupled with SEB (0.25 mg SEB/10 mg sepharose beads) and purified anti Lyt2 mAb (0.5 mg mAb/10 mg sepharose beads). **b** Cell sorter-purified $CD8^+$ responder cells were activated with soluble SEB (10 µg/ml) in the presence of mitomycin (40 µg/ml, 15 min, 37 °C) treated syngeneic LPS blasts (1 × 10⁴/well) (+) or in the presence of mitomycin-treated and glutaraldehyde-fixed (0.16%, 20 min, 37°C) syngeneic LPS blasts (1 × 10⁴/well) (*). The culture period lasted 7 days

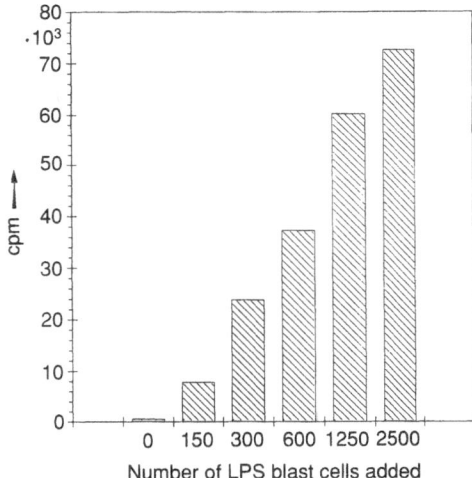

Fig. 4. LPS blast cells provide costimulator activity. Titrated numbers of syngeneic LPS blasts were cocultured together with cell sorter-purified CD8$^+$ T cells (5 × 10^3/well) and immobilized SEB

is cross-linked in addition. A similar conclusion can be drawn from experiments using paraformaldehyde-fixed MHC class II-expressing Lipopolysaccharide (LPS) blast cells as feeder cells. Although these cells bind SEB (as detected by incubation with FITC-coupled SEB and subsequent FACS analysis, data not shown), they do not stimulate resting CD8 T cells to proliferation (Fig. 3b). Since fixed LPS blast cells provide an array of coreceptor ligands (MHC, ICAM) but fail to stimulate resting CD8 T cells, we conclude that primary activation of SEB-reactive T cells is critically dependent on additional costimulator signals delivered by functional APC.

When resting CD8 T cells were stimulated with immobilized SEB the costimulator signal necessary for T cell activation could readily be provided by irradiated syngeneic splenocytes (data not given). Since mAb against MHC class II blocked this response (data not shown), we concluded that class II MHC-expressing splenocytes would be activated via cross-linking of their MHC class II molecules by immobilized SEB, thus gaining the capacity to provide costimulator signals. With this rationale in mind, we tested several in vitro activated cell types for their ability to serve as costimulator cells. We found that irradiated syngeneic LPS blast cells were most effective in providing costimulator signals. As few as 150 LPS blast cells added to CD8 T cells stimulated with immobilized SEB covalently bound to sepharose were sufficient to mount a substantional proliferative response (Fig. 4). Limiting dilution analysis revealed that addition of irradiated syngeneic LPS blasts to CD8 T cells stimulated with immobilized SEB increased the number of proliferating T cell precursors more than 100-fold (from f = 1/2000 to f = 1/20). Control experiments using supernatants from both SEB-coupled beads and syngeneic LPS blast cells preincubated with immobilized SEB to stimulate CD8 T cells excluded the possibility that SEB leaking from SEB-coupled beads was responsible for this effect (MIETHKE et al. 1991). Thus SEB covalently bound to sepharose beads is sufficient to deliver the first signal necessary for primary T cell activation, namely, engagement and cross-linking of TCRs (Fig. 4). However, SEB-induced activation is critically dependent on costimulatory signals provided by activated costimulator cells (Fig. 4) but seems to be independent of cross-linking of the CD8 coreceptors (Figs. 1, 3a).

4 Coreceptor Requirements During Triggering of SEB-Specific Cytotoxic T Lymphocytes

As opposed to conventional antigeneic stimulation, CD8 and CD4 murine T lymphocytes develop into cytolytic effector T cells (CTL) after incubation with soluble SEB and syngeneic feeder cells (HEEG et al. 1991). Using the limiting dilution approach, we found that acquisition of the cytolytic function of murine CD4 T cells is a unique property of superantigen stimulation. In contrast to conventional MHC class II-dependent antigens, after stimulation with SEB every third proliferating CD4 T lymphocyte gained lytic capacity (Table 3), whereas almost every proliferating CD8 T cell developed into a cytolytic progeny (Table 3). However, SEB-reactive CD8 CTL require MHC class II-expressing target cells for triggering of cytolytic responses in the presence of SEB (HERRMANN et al. 1990; FLEISCHER and SCHREZENMEIER 1988), suggesting CD8 coreceptor-independent recognition of SEB on class II MHC-positive target cells. Indeed, addition of anti-CD8 mAb to the cytolytic assay, which almost completely blocks class I MHC-directed cytolysis of CD8 CTL (MACDONALD et al. 1981; HEEG et al. 1990), fails to inhibit CD8-mediated SEB-specific cytolysis (Table 4). Furthermore, xenogeneic human MHC class II- expressing pokeweed mitogen (PWM) blasts were lysed in the presence of SEB by murine SEB-reactive CD8 CTL (Fig. 5), underlining the coreceptor-independent triggering of lytic effector

Table 3. Frequency analysis of SEB-reactive proliferating (PTL-p) and cytolytic (CTL-p) T lymphocyte precursor cells in CD4 and CD8 T lymphocytes

Responder cell	1/PTL-p frequency	1/CTL-p frequency
CD8	22.4	24.0
CD4	34.2	84.3

Cell sorter-purified CD4 or CD8 T lymphocytes were incubated under limiting dilution conditions with 10 µg/ml SEB and irradiated syngeneic feeder cells. After 7 days (CD8 T cells) or 9 days (CD4 T cells) the cultures were split and tested for [^{3}H] thymidine uptake and lytic activity against syngeneic LPS blast target cells in the presence of SEB. From the fraction of negative cultures the frequency was calculated

Table 4. Anti-CD4 or anti-CD8 mAb fail to block the lytic effector function of SEB-reactive CTL

Responder T cell	mAb dilution	Specific lysis (%)
CD4	Anti-L3T4	
	1/50	28
	1/100	31
	1/200	33
	0	35
CD8	Anti-Lyt2	
	1/50	41
	1/100	45
	1/200	50
	0	52

Microcultures of 5000 cell sorter-purified CD4 or CD8 T cells were stimulated with 10 μg/ml SEB; irradiated syngeneic feeder cells; and 10 U/ml recombinant IL-2. After 7 days the cells were harvested and tested in the presence of the indicated mAb against syngeneic LPS blast target cells in the presence of SEB. The % specific lysis at an effector-target ratio of 12:1 is shown

mechanisms. Similar results were obtained with SEB-reactive CD4 CTL: anti-CD4 mAb lack the ability to block the delivery of a lethal hit by CD4 CTL (Table 4). Thus, triggering of the lytic machinery of both SEB-reactive CD8 and CD4 CTL is CD4/CD8 coreceptor-independent but requires MHC-class II expression on the target cells.

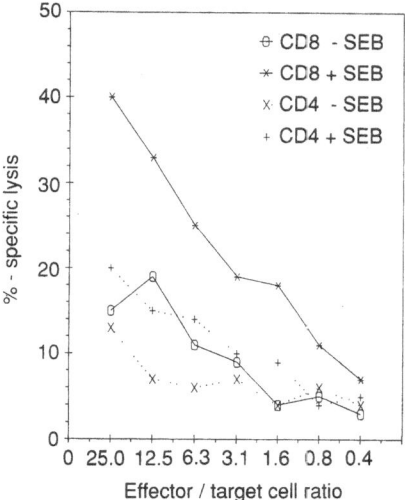

Fig. 5. Murine SEB-reactive CTL recognize xenogeneic target cells in the presence of SEB. Populations of 5000 cell sorter-purified CD4 and CD8 T lymphocytes were cultured with SEB and syngeneic feeder cells. After 7 days, cells were harvested and assayed in a ^{51}Cr release assay against human pokeweed mitogen (PWM) blast target cells in the presence or absence of SEB ⊖, CD8-SEB; ∗, CD8 + SEB; ×, CD4-SEB; +, CD4 + SEB

5 Coreceptor Requirements During SEB-Mediated Negative Selection of $V_\beta 8$-Expressing Thymocytes

Injection of SEB into newborn mice effectively prevents the maturation of $V_\beta 8$-expressing peripheral T cells (WHITE et al. 1989; JENKINSON et al. 1989). Obviously double positive (DP) CD4 + CD8 + thymocytes recognize SEB bound to MHC class II-expressing thymic cells and become clonally deleted (WHITE et al. 1989) resulting in a lack of peripheral $V_\beta 8$-expressing CD4 and CD8 T lymphocytes (WHITE et al. 1989). To test whether the SEB- mediated negative selection of $V_\beta 8$ thymocytes is dependent on engagement of the CD4 coreceptor of DP thymocytes with class II MHC molecules of thymic cells presenting SEB, we injected anti-CD4 mAb in addition to SEB into newborn mice. The injection of anti-CD4 mAb into newborn mice was reported to block effectively the maturation of single positive (SP) CD4+ thymocytes, presumably by hindering CD4-MHC class II interactions necessary for positive selection (ZUNIGA-PFLUCKER et al. 1989; VON BOEHMER 1988). As can be seen in Fig. 6, injection of anti-CD4 mAb prevented the selection of SP CD4 thymocytes, suggesting an effective blockade of the CD4-MHC class II interaction, but had no effect on CD8 maturation (Fig. 6b). However, upon coinjection of SEB, $V_\beta 8$-expressing CD8 thymocytes were still deleted (Fig. 6f). Therefore, we conclude that SEB-mediated clonal deletion of V_β- expressing thymocytes is independent of CD4-MHC class II interactions.

6 Conclusion

Activation and triggering of conventional T lymphocytes recognizing peptides bound to MHC molecules are critically dependent on CD4 or CD8 coreceptors (BIERER et al. 1989). CD4 or CD8 coreceptors associate specifically with constant regions of the MHC class II or MHC class I molecules, respectively (DOYLE and STROMINGER 1987; NORMENT et al. 1988). This further strengthens complex formation between CD3-TCR and antigen-presenting MHC molecule and provides additional intracellular signals via CD4/8-associated $p56^{lck}$ tyrosine kinase activity (VEILLETTE et al. 1988, 1989). The adhesion function of this interaction was clearly demonstrated using T cell lines transfected with CD4/8 molecules lacking the intracytoplasmic domain responsible for $p56^{lck}$ binding (SLECKMAN et al. 1988; ZAMOYSKA et al. 1989). Morevoer, the failure of murine T lymphocytes to recognize at high frequency human MHC xenoantigens or antigens bound to human MHC molecules could be reversed by transfection of human CD8 coreceptors into murine T lymphocytes expressing HLA-specific TCRs (ARNOLD, personal communication). The adhesion function of the CD4/8 molecules seems to be obligate for triggering the majority of antigen-specific T

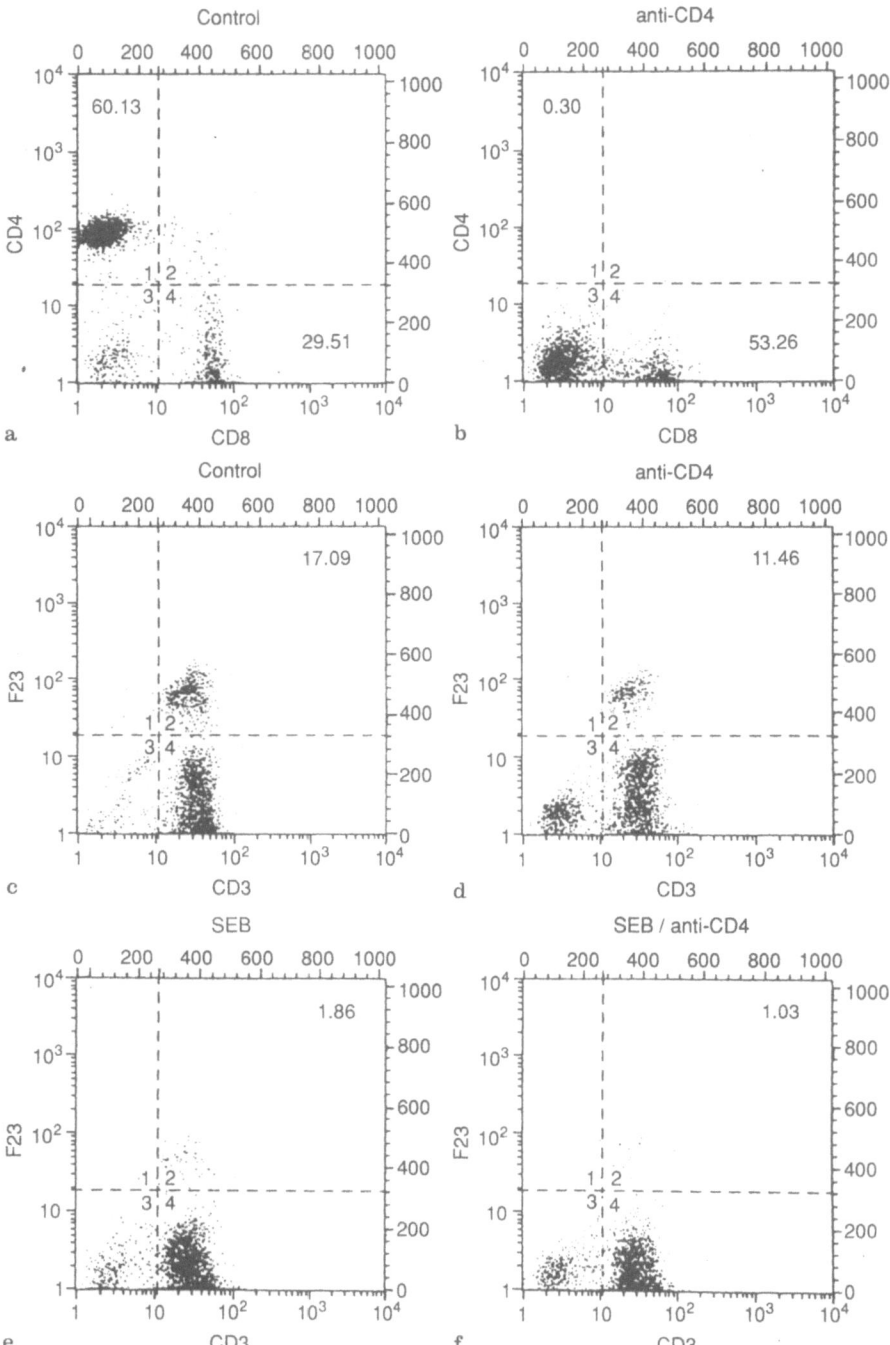

Fig. 6a–f. Thymic deletion of $V_\beta 8$-expressing T cells is independent of CD4 coreceptors. Newborn B6 mice were injected with anti-CD4 mAb (**b, d**), SEB (**e**), or a combination of both (**f**). After 7 days, mice received hydrocortisone to enrich for mature thymocytes. Thymocytes were stained with FITC-conjugated anti-CD8 mAb (**a, b**) or FITC-conjugated anti-CD3 mAb (**c–f**) and PE-conjugated anti-CD4 mAb (**a, b**) or biotin-coupled anti-$V_\beta 8$ mAb (F23) followed by streptavidin-PE; 3×10^4 gated cells were analyzed cytofluorometrically

cells (BIERER et al. 1989; SPRENT et al. 1986; MIZUOCHI et al. 1986; HEEG et al. 1987). However, the intracellular signals provided by cross-linked CD4/8 molecules do not appear to be essential but rather enhance T cell triggering as shown by transfection of truncated CD4/8 genes (SLECKMAN et al. 1988; ZAMOYSKA et al. 1989) or by stimulating T cells with suboptimal concentrations of anti- α/β or anti-CD3 mAb (EICHMANN et al. 1987).

In contrast, recognition of the superantigen SEB is independent of CD4/8 coreceptors. This conclusion is based on the following observations: (a) SEB bound to MHC class II molecules is effectively and at high frequency recognized by CD8 T lymphocytes (Fig. 1, Table 1); (b) primary activation of SEB-reactive T cells cannot be blocked by anti-CD8 mAb (Fig. 1); (c) triggering of lytic effector mechanisms does not require CD4 or CD8 molecules (Table 4); (d) xenogeneic blast cells are lysed by SEB-reactive CD8 CTL (Fig. 5), indicating the independence of species–specific CD4/8-MHC interactions); and (e) thymic negative selection of $V_\beta 8$-expressing T lymphocytes is not blocked by anti-CD4 mAb (Fig. 6). However, in the presence of sufficient costimulator activity, CD8 cross-linking enhances the proliferative response of resting CD8 T cells stimulated with SEB (Fig. 1). In contrast to stimulation with suboptimal amounts of anti-α/β or CD3 mAb (EICHMANN et al. 1987; KOSSIK, personal communication), CD8 cross-linking is not able to substitute for the costimulator activity necessary for primary T cell activation of SEB-reactive T lymphocytes (Fig. 3a). The observations that CD8 T cells respond to a variety of exogenous superantigens when presented by MHC class II molecules suggest that this might be a general rule for superantigen recognition (HERRMANN et al. 1990; HEEG et al. 1991). Indeed, endogenous superantigens such as Mls (JANEWAY et al. 1989) also effectively stimulate CD8 T lymphocytes (WEBB and SPRENT 1990; MACDONALD et al. 1990). However, the role of CD4/8 molecules in determining the functional phenotype of superantigen-reactive T lymphocytes is as yet unresolved. It is striking that, in contrast to stimulation with conventional antigens, murine SEB-reactive CD4 T cells gain powerful lytic effector capacity (Tables 3 and 4); so far no Mls-reactive CD8 CTL have been reported (WEBB and SPRENT 1990; MACDONALD et al. 1990).

According to the two signal concept of T cell activation (BRETSCHER and COHN 1970; SCHWARTZ 1990), primary activation of T cells is dependent on recognition of antigen by the TCR-CD3 complex (signal 1) and on TCR-unlinked costimulatory signals provided by functional APC (signal 2). Antigens presented by APC not capable of delivering the costimulator signal do not activate but rather anergize the responding T cells (SCHWARTZ 1989, 1990; JENKINS et al. 1988; GASPARI et al. 1988). T cell activation by SEB seems to fit this concept. SEB bound to sepharose beads or to APC fixed with paraformaldehyde failed to stimulate SEB-reactive T cells (Fig. 2, Fig. 3b). Even co-cross-linking of CD8 molecules did not restore the ability of sepharose-conjugated SEB to induce T cell proliferation (Fig. 3a). In our hands, irradiated LPS blast cells were effective in providing the obligatory costimulator signal: as few as 150 LPS blast cells converted unresponsive T cells stimulated with sepharose-bound SEB to a proliferative response (Fig. 4). Whether $V_\beta 8$ T cells become clonally silenced by immobilized

SEB is currently being investigated. Recently, similar conclusions were drawn with human T cells stimulated with immobilized superantigen streptococcal M protein (TOMAI et al. 1990). Although soluble M protein was sufficient to trigger human T cells to proliferation on feeder cells, it failed to activate T lymphocytes when immobilized in the absence of feeder cells (KOTB et al. 1990). This failure could be overcome by adding phorbol esters, thus providing an intracellular costimulator signal (KOTB et al. 1990). Hence, TCR- unlinked costimulator signals seem to be essential for primary activation of superantigen-reactive T cells.

Taken together, triggering of T lymphocytes with the superantigen SEB differs from activation with conventional antigens. Recognition of unprocessed SEB requires binding to MHC class II molecules, yet is CD4/8 coreceptor-independent. Unlinked to their CD4/CD8 phenotype, T lymphocytes with the appropriate V_β-bearing TCR become triggered. However, primary activation of SEB-reactive T cells depends critically on TCR-unlinked costimulator signals provided by functional APC.

Acknowledgements. We thank Mrs. Birgit Deeg and Susanne Hausmann for their excellent technical help.

References

Bierer BE, Sleckman BP, Ratnofsky SE, Burakoff SJ (1989) The biologic roles of CD2, CD4, and CD8 in T-cell activation. Annu Rev Immunol 7: 579–599

Bjorkman PJ, Saper MA, Samraour B, Bennet WS, Strominger JL, Wiley DC (1987) The foreign antigen binding site and T cell recognition regions of class I histocompatibility antigens. Nature 329: 506–512

Bretscher P, Cohn M (1970) A theory of self-nonself discrimination. Science 169: 1042–1044

Buus S, Sette A, Colon SM, Miles C, Grey HM (1987) The relation between major histocompatibility complex (MHC) restriction and the capacity of Ia to bind immunogenic peptides. Science 235:1353–1358

Choi YW, Herman A, DiGiusto D, Wade T, Marrack P, Kappler J (1990) Residues of the variable region of the T cell receptor beta-chain that interact with S. aureus toxin superantigens. Nature 346: 471–473

Davis MM, Bjorkman PJ (1988) T-cell antigen receptor genes and T-cell recognition. Nature 334: 395–402

Doyle C, Strominger JL (1987) Interaction between CD4 and class II MHC molecules mediates cell adhesion. Nature 330: 256–259

Eichmann K, Jönsson J-I, Falk I, Emmrich F (1987) Effective activation of resting mouse T lymphocytes by cross-linking submitogenic concentration of the T cell antigen receptor with either Lyt2 or L3T4. Eur J Immunol 17: 643–650

Fischer H, Dohlsten M, Lindvall M, Sjogren HO, Carlsson R (1989) Binding of staphylococcal enterotoxin A to HLA-DR on B cell lines. J Immunol 142: 3151–3157

Fleischer B, Schrezenmeier H (1988) T cell stimulation by staphylococcal enterotoxins. Clonally variable response and requirement for major histocompatibility complex class II molecules on accessory or target cells. J Exp Med 167: 1697–1707

Fleischer B, Schrezenmeier H, Conradt P (1989) T lymphocyte activation by staphylococcal enterotoxins: role of class II molecules and T cell surface structures. Cell Immunol 120: 92–101

Fraser JD (1989) High-affinity binding of staphylococcal enterotoxins A and B to HLA-DR. Nature 339: 221–223

Gaspari AA, Jenkins MK, Katz SI (1988) Class II MHC-bearing keratinocytes induce antigen-specific unresponsiveness in hapten-specific Th1 clones. J Immunol 141: 2216–2220

Geppert TD, Davis LS, Gur H, Wacholtz MC, Lipsky PE (1990) Accessory cell signals involved in T-cell activation. Immunol Rev 117: 5–66

Heeg K, Steeg C, Schmitt J, Wagner H (1987) Frequency analysis of class I MHC-reactive Lyt2[+] and class II MHC-reactive L3T4[+] IL-2-secreting T lymphocytes. J Immunol 138: 4121–4127

Heeg K, Bendigs S, Bader P, Miethke T, Wagner H (1991) Reactivity of murine T cell subsets against the superantigen SEB: identification of high frequent, high affinity, and MHC unrestricted cytotoxic T cell precursors in CD8[+] and CD4[+] T cells. (submitted)

Herrmann T, Accolla RS, MacDonald HR (1989) Different staphylococcal enterotoxins bind preferentially to distinct major histocompatibility complex class II isotypes. Eur J Immunol 19: 2171–2174

Herrmann T, Maryanski JL, Romero P, Fleischer B, MacDonald HR (1990) Activation of MHC-class I restricted CD8[fA074] CTL by microbial T cell mitogens. Dependence upon MHC class II expression on the target cells and V_β usage of the responder T cells. J Immunol 144: 1181–1186

Janeway CA, Chalupny J, Conrad PJ, Buxser S (1988) An external stimulus that mimics Mls locus responses. J Immunogenet 15: 161–168

Janeway CA, Yagi J, Conrad PJ, Katz ME, Jones B, Vroegop S, Buxser S (1989) T cell responses to Mls and to bacterial proteins that mimic its behaviour. Immunol Rev 107: 61–88

Jenkins MK, Ashwell JD, Schwartz RH (1988) Allogeneic non-T spleen cells estore the responsiveness of normal T cell clones stimulated with antigen and chemically modified antigen presenting cells. J Immunol 140: 3324–3330

Jenkinson E-J, Knigston R, Smith CA, Williams GT, Owen JJ (1989) Antigen- induced apoptosis in developing T cells: a mechanism for negative selection of the T cell receptor repertoire. Eur J Immunol 19: 2175–2177

Kappler J, Kotzin B, Herron L, Gelfand EW, Bigler RD, Boylston A, Carrel S, Posnett DN, Choi Y, Marrach P (1989) V beta-specific stimulation of human T cells by staphylococcal toxins. Science 244: 811–813

Karp DR, Teletski CL, Scholl P, Geha R, Long EO (1990) The alpha 1 domain of the HLA-DR molecule is essential for high-affinity binding of the toxic shock syndrome toxin-1. Nature 346: 474–476

Kaye J, Porcelli S, Tite J, Jones B, Janeway CA Jr (1983) Both monoclonal antibody and antisera specific for determinants unique to individual cloned helper T cell lines can substitute for antigen and antigen-presenting cells in the activation of T cells. J Exp Med 158: 836–856

Kotb M, Majumdar G, Tomai M, Beachey EH (1990) Accessory cell- independent stimulation of human T cells by streptococcal M protein superantigen. J Immunol 145: 1332–1336

MacDonald HR, Thiernesse N, Cerottini JC (1981) Inhibition of T-cell mediated cytolysis by monoclonal antibodies directed against Lyt2: heterogeneity of inhibition at the clonal level. J Immunol 126: 1671–1675

MacDonald HR, Lees RK, Chvatchko Y (1990) CD8[+] T cells respond clonally to Mls- 1[a]-encoded determinants. J Exp Med 171: 1381–1386

Marrack P, Kappler J (1990) The Staphylococcal enterotoxins and their relatives. Science 248: 1066

Matis LA (1990) The molecular basis of T cell specificity. Annu Rev Immunol 8: 65–82

Meuer SC, Hussey RE, Cantrell DA, Hodgon DC, Schlossman SF, Smith KA, Reinherz EL (1984a) Triggering of the T3-Ti antigen receptor complex results in clonal T cell proliferation through an interleukin 2-dependent autocrine pathway. Proc Natl Acad Sci USA 81: 1509–1513

Meuer SC, Hussey RE, Fabbi M, Fox D, Acuto O, Fitzgerald KA, Hodgdon JC, Protentis JP, Schlossman SF, Reinherz EL (1984b) An alternative pathway of T-cell activation: a functional role for the 50 kd T11 sheep erythrocyte receptor protein. Cell 36: 897–906

Miethke T, Heeg K, Wahl C, Wagner H (1991) Crosslinked staphylococcal enterotoxin B stimulates CD8[+] T cells only in the presence of unlinked costimulator signals. Immunobiology (in press)

Mizuochi T, Ono S, Malek TR, Sniger A (1986) Characterization of two distinct primary T cell populations that secrete interleukin-2 upon recognition of class I or class II major histocompatibility antigens. J Exp Med 163: 603–619

Mollick JA, Cook RG, Rich RR (1989) Class II MHC molecules are specific receptors for staphylococcus enterotoxin A. Science 244: 817–820

Norment AM, Salter RD, Parham P, Engelhard VM, Littman DR (1988) Cell–cell adhesion mediated by CD8 and MHC class I molecules. Nature 336: 79–81

Russell JK, Pontzer CH, Johnson HM (1990) THe IA beta b region (65-85) is a binding site for the superantigen, staphylococcal enterotoxin A. Biochem Biophys Res Commun 168: 696–701

Scholl PR, Diez A, Geha RS (1989a) Staphylococcal enterotoxin B and toxic shock syndrome toxin-1 bind to distinct sites on HLA-DR and HLA-DQ molecules. J Immunol 143: 2583–2588

Scholl P, Diez A, Mourad W, Parsonnet J, Geha RS, Chatila T (1989b) Toxic shock syndrome toxin-1 binds to major histocompatibility complex class II molecules. Proc Natl Acad Sci USA 86: 4210–4214

Scholl PR, Diez A, Karr R, Sekaly RP, Trowsdale J, Geha RS (1990) Effect of isotypes and allelic polymorphism on the binding staphylococcal enterotoxins to MHC class II molecules. J Immunol 144: 226–230

Schwartz RH (1989) Acquisition of immunologic self-tolerance. Cell 57: 1073–1081

Schwartz RH (1990) A cell culture model for T lymphocyte clonal anergy. Science 248: 1349–1356

Sleckman BP, Peterson A, Foran JA, Gorga JC, Kara CJ, Strominger JL, Burakoff SJ, Greenstein JL (1988) Functional analysis of a cytoplasmic domain-deleted mutant of the CD4 molecule. J Immunol 141: 49–54

Sprent J, Schaefer M, Lo D, Korngold R (1986) Functions of purified L3T4 + and Lyt2 + cells in vitro and in vivo. Immunol Rev 91: 195–218

Staunton DE, Dustin ML, Springer TA (1989) Functional cloning of ICAM-2, a cell adhesion ligand for LFA-1 homologous to ICAM-1. Nature 339: 61–64

Swain SL (1983) T cell subsets and the recognition of MHC class. Immunol Rev 74: 129–142

Tomai M, Kotb M, Majumdar G, Beachey EH (1990) Superantigenicity of streptococcal M protein. J Exp Med 172: 359–362

Townsend AR, Rothbard J, Gotch FM, Bahadur G, Wraith D, McMichael AJ (1986) The epitopes of influenza nucleoprotein recognized by cytotoxic T lymphocytes can be defined with short synthetic peptides. Cell 44: 959–968

Veillette A, Bookman MA, Horak EM, Bolen JB (1988) The CD4 and CD8 T cell surface antigens are associated with the internal membrane tyrosin-protein kinase p56. Cell 55: 301–308

Veillette A, Bookman MA, Horak EM, Samelson LE, Bolen JB (1989) Signal transduction through the CD4 receptor involves the activation of the internal membrane tyrosine-protein kinase p56. Nature 338: 257–259

Webb SR, Sprent J (1990) Response of mature unprimed CD8[+] T cells to Mls[a] determinants. J Exp Med 171: 953–958

White J, Herman AM, Pullen AM, Kubo R, Kappler JW, Marrack P (1989) The V_β-specific superantigen staphylococcal enterotoxin B: stimulation of mature T cells and clonal deletion in neonatal mice. Cell 56: 27–35

Yagi J, Baron J, Baxser S, Janeway CA Jr (1990) Bacterial proteins that mediate the association of a defined subset of T cell receptor: CD4 complexes with class II MHC. J Immunol 144: 892–901

Zamoyska R, Derham P, Gorman SD, von Hoegen P, Bolen JB, Veillette A, Parnes JR (1989) Inability of CD8 alpha' polypeptides to associate with p56[lck] correlates with impaired function in vitro and lack of expression in vivo. Nature 342: 278–281

Zuniga-Pflucker JC, McCarthy SA, Weston M, Longo DL, Sniger A, Kruisbeek AM (1989) Role of CD4 in thymocyte selection and maturation. J Exp Med 169: 2085–2096

The Immunobiology of *Mycoplasma arthritidis* and its Superantigen MAM

B. C. COLE

1 Introduction

A commonly held hypothesis is that the chronic autoimmune rheumatoid diseases of humans are mediated or initiated by infectious agents. It has recently been postulated that "superantigens" might play a role in the development of these autoimmune diseases by activating preexisting anti-self T cells (MARRACK and KAPPLER 1988) and by inducing polyclonal B cell activation leading to the production of autoantibodies (TUMANG et al. 1990). Of special interest is the superantigen MAM (*Mycoplasma arthritidis* T cell mitogen) which is produced by a microorganism that is known to cause a chronic relapsing arthritis in rodents.

Mycoplasmas are the most common cause of naturally occurring acute and chronic arthritis in many animal species. In fact, early work on mycoplasma-induced murine arthritis led Sabin to propose in 1939 that these organisms might be the etiological agents of human rheumatoid arthritis. Despite reports describing the isolation of mycoplasmas from human rheumatoid tissues, the vast majority of investigators have failed to corroborate these findings. However, there are numerous reports describing the ability of human- specific species of mycoplasma to invade the joints of immunocompromised patients. Furthermore,

Division of Rheumatology, Department of Internal Medicine, University of Utah School of Medicine, 50 North Medical Drive, Salt Lake City, UT 84132, USA

acute or chronic joint disease can be a late complication of *M. pneumoniae* infection (see reviews by CASSELL and COLE 1981; COLE et al. 1985b).

In this review, I will summarize current knowledge on the properties of MAM and its interaction with cells of the immune system in vitro and in vivo and will discuss its role in both acute and chronic disease mediated by *M. arthritidis.*

2 Properties of MAM

As reviewed earlier (COLE et al. 1985b), MAM was first detected during studies to determine the role of cell-mediated immune responses in the development of *M. arthritidis*-induced arthritis of mice. Both normal lymphocytes and lymphocytes from arthritic mice were shown to undergo proliferation in response to both sonified mycoplasma cell antigens and to viable organisms. Subsequently, cell-free culture supernatants of *M. arthritidis* were shown to induce cytolytic lymphocytes and lymphocyte proliferation (COLE et al. 1981). The mitogenic component of mycoplasma cells was stable to 100°C and was active only for B lymphocytes. In contrast, the soluble component in culture supernatants was shown to be heat labile and was active for T lymphocytes. Whereas B cell mitogens are present in the membranes of many species of mycoplasmas, a soluble T cell mitogen has so far been isolated only from *M. arthritidis.*

Lymphocyte activation by *M. arthritidis* supernatants also results in induction of interferon-γ (IFN-γ) (COLE and THORPE 1984; KIRCHNER et al. 1984) and interleukin-2) (IL-2) (YOWELL et al. 1983). In addition, *M. arthritidis* cells and supernatants activated a macrophage cell line resulting in increased listericidal and tumoricidal properties (DIETZ and COLE 1982). More recent studies using partially purified MAM have demonstrated induction of granulocyte/macrophage colony-stimulating factor (GM-CSF) by human peripheral blood mononuclear cells (NAOT and COLE, unpublished observations). Membranes from *M. arthritidis* have also been shown to induce GM-CSF in murine bone marrow-derived macrophages (STUART et al. 1990).

MAM is produced to maximal titer in senescent broth cultures of *M. arthritidis.* Purification has been difficult due to the paucity of material produced and to its heat lability and affinity for glass and plastic surfaces as well as to large molecules present in mycoplasma culture media. The mitogen is a heat (56°C) and acid (< pH 7.0) labile protein with an unusually high pI of > 9.0 (ATKIN et al. 1986).

Homogeneous preparations have recently been obtained by a complex purification scheme involving $(NH_4)_2SO_4$ fractionation followed by gel filtration chromatography, two cation exchanges, and finally hydrophobic interaction chromatography (ATKIN et al., unpublished observations). MAM prepared in this way has a molecular weight of approximately 27 000 by gel electrophoresis.

A comparison of the sequence of the first 54 amino acids of MAM with the sequences of the staphylococcal superantigens fails to identify any common epitopes. Furthermore, no significant homology has been identified between MAM and any of the protein sequences in the gene bank and the National Biomedical Research Foundation computer libraries (OLIPHANT et al., unpublished observations). Thus, the present fragment of MAM appears to be unique. MAM is extraordinary potent, giving 50% of the maximal proliferative response of murine lymphocytes at $< 10^{-14} M$ (ATKIN et al., unpublished observations).

3 Activation of Mouse Lymphocytes by MAM

Detailed descriptions of murine T cell activation by MAM are reviewed elsewhere (COLE 1988; COLE and ATKIN 1991). Only the main issues will be described here.

The serendipitous finding was made that lymphocytes from C57BL/10 mice failed to undergo proliferation in response to MAM, whereas those from BALB/c and C3H mice were readily activated. The negative or weak response of the C57BL/10 mice was used as a marker which enabled the gene which controls MAM reactivity to be mapped to the I-E region of the murine H2 major histocompatibility complex (MHC) (COLE et al. 1981). This observation was consistent with the fact that MAM-induced T cell proliferation was dependent upon MHC-bearing accessory cells (AC) (COLE et al. 1982b). This specificity for I-E bearing cells suggested that the I-E molecule might be a binding site for MAM. It was subsequently shown using congenic and recombinant mouse strains that only splenocytes from I-E-bearing mouse strains could remove MAM activity from solution (COLE et al. 1982a). Unlike the presentation of antigen to T cells by AC, the presentation of MAM required neither processing nor an IL-1 signal (COLE et al. 1986a). Later work showed that liposomes with incorporated I-E but not with I-A molecules could also present MAM to T cells (BEKOFF et al. 1987).

There is substantial evidence that the conserved α chain of the I-E molecule, or a combinatorial determinant between E_α and other β chains, bears the MAM receptor since: (1) ATFR5 mice which lack E_β respond to MAM via combinatorial $E_\alpha A_\beta$ molecules; (2) antibody to a MAb specific for E_α totally blocks MAM-induced proliferation; (3) E_α transgenic mice on a C57BL/10 background present MAM; and (4) transfected fibroblasts expressing $E_\alpha E_\beta$ or $E_\alpha A_\beta$ present MAM, whereas fibroblasts expressing $A_\alpha A_\beta$ do not (COLE et al. 1990a).

T cell recognition of MAM is not MHC-restricted since T cells need not recognize self MHC as long as the AC bear the I-E molecule (COLE and ATKIN 1991; YOWELL et al. 1983). Furthermore, T cell responses are clonally expressed. In one study, only 6 of 34 T cell lines responded to MAM irrespective of CD4 or CD8 expression (LYNCH et al. 1986).

It was recently shown that, as for other superantigens, MAM is recognized by the V_β chains of the α/β T cell receptor for antigen (TCR) (COLE et al. 1989,

1990b). This was demonstrated using the RIIIS mouse which exhibits massive deletions in its $V_\beta \alpha/\beta$ T cell repertoire (HAQQI et al. 1989) and the B10.RIII mouse which retains all V_β genes. In RIIIS test-cross progeny with (RIIIS × B10.RIII)F1 hybrids, reactivity of lymphocytes with MAM cosegregated with expression of $V_\beta 8$-bearing cells as detected by immunofluorescence. Clonal expansion of MAM-reactive BALB/c cells in vitro followed by immunofluorescence showed that activated cells expressed $V_\beta 8.1$, $V_\beta 8.2$, $V_\beta 8.3$, or $V_\beta 6$, with $V_\beta 8.2$-bearing cells predominating at 46.2% of the total; in contrast, $V_\beta 6$-bearing cells represented only 6.7% of the total. MAM expansion of C57BR lymphocytes which lack the $V_\beta 8$ genes resulted in a 61% expression of $V_\beta 6$ in the activated population (COLE et al. 1990b). Since none of the percentages add up to 100%, it seems likely that MAM can use other V_β TCRs. It is of interest that, whereas usage of products of the $V_\beta 8$ TCR gene family is fairly common amongst other microbial superantigens, $V_\beta 6$ is only used by MAM and by the Mls 1^a self antigen (KAPPLER et al. 1988; MACDONALD et al. 1988).

4 Activation of Human T and B Cells by MAM

Previous work had established that MAM could also activate human T cells and that this reaction was also dependent upon MHC- bearing AC (COLE et al. 1982c; DAYNES et al. 1982). In this case, the human HLA-DR MHC molecule, which is the equivalent of the murine I-E molecule (and structurally closely related), appears to possess the binding site for MAM, since anti-HLA.DR antibodies inhibited proliferation, IFN-γ production, and the induction of cytolytic cells in response to MAM (COLE and THORPE 1983; MATTHES et al. 1988). Furthermore, cells transfected with I-E can present MAM to human T cells and the response is inhibitable with the anti-I-E monoclonal antibody (mAb), 14.4.4s (MATTHES et al. 1988).

In an analysis of the reactivity of a wide range of human T cell clones to MAM, it was shown that MAM could induce proliferation or cytotoxicity irrespective of expression of the CD4 or CD8 molecules. TCR α/β-negative, γ/δ-positive cells also respond to MAM in the presence of appropriate AC. Although full activation of T cells fails to occur in the absence of AC, an increase in cytoplasmic Ca^{2+} concentrations can be detected. In addition, phorbol myristate acetate, which is an activator of protein kinase C, could induce T cell proliferation in the absence of AC. These observations led to the proposal that MAM might be a bivalent molecule which can interact separately with TCRs and MHC molecules (MATTHES et al. 1988).

In a number of studies, the response of human cells to MAM has always been found to be less than the response seen with mouse cells and less than the response to lectin mitogens (COLE et al. 1982c; CANNON et al. 1986). Recently, a direct comparison was made between the responses of MAM and other microbial superantigens to activate murine vs human lymphocytes. Human cells clearly responded better to staphylococcal superantigens than to MAM and murine cells responded better to MAM (FLEISCHER et al. 1991). This difference appears to be due to differences in the MHC/superantigen interaction since lymphocytes from transgenic mice expressing human MHC molecules respond better to the staphylococcal superantigens than to MAM (COLE et al., unpublished observations).

The ability of superantigens to interact with both MHC molecules on AC and B cells and V_β TCRs on T cells raises the possibility that these substances might be able to initiate a B-T_H cell collaboration resulting in polyclonal B cell activation. Preliminary evidence of B cell activation by MAM came from the observation that peripheral blood lymphocytes from normal individuals or rheumatoid arthritis (RA) patients secreted significantly higher levels of IgG when co-cultured in vitro with MAM and pokeweed mitogen. In addition, low levels of IgM rheumatoid factor (RF) were secreted by lymphocytes from normal or seronegative RA patients (EMERY et al. 1985).

To more specifically address this issue, MAM-reactive T_H cell lines were generated by in vitro exposure of peripheral blood monocytes to MAM, separation of T blasts by gradient centrifugation, and selection of T_H cells by immune rosette depletion of CD8$^+$ cells. Purified B cell cultures, or B cells incubated with MAM-reactive T_H Cells, failed to secrete significant levels of IgM. However, when the B cells were pulsed with MAM and washed or when MAM was added to the B-T_H cell mixture high levels of IgM (6-7 ng/ml) were produced. Similar observations were made using resting tonsillar B lymphocytes (TUMANG et al. 1990).

The importance of these observations is that the abnormal T_H-B cell interaction mimics that seen in graft vs host disease which has been used as a model to study systemic lupus erythematosus. In the latter chronic systemic disease, abnormal B cell reactivity results in the production of a wide range of autoantibodies, especially to antigens on cell surfaces such as lymphocytes and to antigens with repetitive sequences such as DNA (FRIEDMAN et al. 1991).

5 Activation of Rat T Cells by MAM

Mycoplasma arthritidis causes a severe suppurative arthritis in rats, and the disease can also be associated with conjunctivitis, urethritis, lethargy, and paralysis (WARD and JONES 1962) and, more recently, uveitis (THIRKILL and GREGERSON 1982). Rat lymphocytes can also be activated by the MAM superantigen (COLE et al. 1982c). A comparison of splenic cells from various inbred rat strains indicated that DA, Lewis, Buffalo, August, Wistar Furth, and (LEW x BN)F1 all responded well to MAM, phytohemagglutinin, and concanavalin A, but cells from BN and MAXX rats were very weakly or nonresponsive to all mitogens. Cells from congenic strains expressing nonresponder background genes and responder haplotypes at RT1 failed to respond significantly to the mitogens (MORITZ et al. 1984; COLE et al. 1986b). Rats expressing responder background genes but the nonresponder haplotype at RT1 exhibited high responses to all mitogens. The controlling role of non-RT1 genes was confirmed by testing tissue-typed (DA × BN)F2 progeny for lymphocyte reactivity to MAM. No association was seen between the expression of responder vs nonresponder haplotypes at RT1 and the degree of response to the mitogens. In contrast, as the proportion of DA non-RT1 genes increased, so did the degree of mitogenic responsiveness (COLE et al. 1986b). The results indicated that in the (DA × BN)F1 hybrids, responsiveness to all mitogens was recessive: this contrasts with the (LEW × BN)F1 hybrids in which responsiveness was dominant. Both responder and nonresponder splenic cells were capable of binding the *M. arthritidis* mitogen. The data contrast with those obtained with nonresponder mouse strains, the cells of which failed to bind mitogen due to the absence of the E_α chain of the I-E-coded molecule. The results clearly indicate that a distinct gene is responsible for the failure of BN lymphocytes to respond to T cell mitogens. It remains to be determined whether this hyporeactive response relates to rat V_β TCR expression.

It is of great interest that the genetics of MAM-induced activation of rat lymphocytes closely resemble that seen for susceptibility to two different experimentally induced autoimmune diseases. Thus, (LEW × BN)F1 rats are susceptible to experimental allergic encephalomyelitis (EAE) and collagen-induced arthritis, whereas (DA × BN)F1 rats are resistant (GRIFFITHS and DEWITT 1984; GASSER et al. 1973). More work is required to identify the mechanism for these differences. Recent work indicates that in both of these autoimmune diseases T cells expressing $V_\beta 8$ TCRs are involved in disease pathogenesis. Since the rat and mouse V_β TCRs are quite similar, it is likely that MAM also activates rat $V_\beta 8$-bearing T cells.

6 Pathogenicity of *Mycoplasma arthritidis* and its Superantigen MAM

The ability of an infectious agent to invade the naive host and to initiate and perpetuate disease is dependent upon a complex interplay between the specific attributes of the agent and their interactions with the immune response of the host. The mycoplasmas are a very successful group of parasites which associate closely with the cells of their hosts. They are the causative agents of respiratory, genitourinary, and joint diseases of animals and humans (RAZIN and BARILE 1985). The chronicity of many of these diseases and the apparent difficulty of the host in eliminating these organisms suggest a unique ability to bypass or evade host defense mechanisms. *Mycoplasma arthritidis* illustrates these properties very well and this subject is reviewed in more detail elsewhere (COLE et al. 1985b). The effect of MAM on this host/parasite interaction is discussed below.

6.1 Immunosuppression and Invasion of the Host

Mycoplasma arthritidis is frequently harbored in the respiratory tract of apparently healthy animals. Its presence may be difficult to detect unless extensive culturing is performed since an antibody response may not be present (DAVIDSON et al. 1983). The environmental factors which determine the development of spontaneous disease are poorly understood.

Despite the rapid onset of complement-fixing (CF) antibodies after experimental injection of organisms, there is strong evidence that the immune response to *M. arthritidis* is defective. Neutralizing or growth inhibiting antibodies, which play a major role in the control of mycoplasma infections, are not produced against *M. arthritidis* in rodents. Furthermore, opsonizing antibodies are likewise not evoked. It is not surprising, therefore, that a myco-plasmemia persists in the peripheral circulation for up to 3 weeks following IV injection of the organisms (COLE et al. 1985b). MAM production by these organisms may be responsible for the depressed host defenses. As an example, mycoplasmas are cleared faster from the peripheral circulation of mouse strains which lack a functional I-E molecules (C3H-SW) than they are from strains possessing I-E (C3H) (COLE et al. 1983).

In addition, the systemic injection of mice with high doses of MAM results in a state of anergy in which T cells from treated animals lose much of their ability to proliferate in vitro in response to MAM, the staphylococcal superantigen SEB, and, to a somewhat lesser extent, to Con A and PHA (COLE and WELLS 1990). This anergic state is due to an MAM-activated, CD4-positive T cell which can suppress the response of normal T cells to mitogens. This response appears limited to mouse strains which express a functional I-E molecule and, presum-ably, to mouse strains which bear the appropriate MAM-reactive V_β TCRs. The mechanism of this suppressive effect remains to be established. However, there is evidence that viable cells are required for transfer of suppression in vitro. Although transfer of suppression is not MHC-restricted, there are indications that it might be V_β α/β TCR-restricted. Thus, mice injected with MAM respond normally to SEA, and lymphocytes from mice injected with SEA fail to respond to SEA but show only slight inhibition of responses to MAM (COLE and AHMED, unpublished observations).

We have also shown that a series of injections of MAM before and during skin grafts slightly but significantly prolongs graft survival. Furthermore, MAM, given prior to sensitization with dinitrofluorobenzene, partially suppresses the development of contact sensitivity. If suppression of immune reactivity of T cells is indeed V_β-specific, then the degree of suppression of graft rejections and contact sensitivity must be limited by T cells bearing $V_\beta 6$ and $V_\beta 8$ TCRs.

Somewhat variable results have been obtained when MAM is given prior to antigenic challenge with foreign proteins or sheep red blood cells. However, if MAM is given at the same time as, or particularly, after antigen administration, then antibody responses are increased (COLE and AHMED, unpublished obser-vations). These observations are consistent with the polyclonal B cell activation by MAM described earlier. It would seem from these preliminary studies that time of administration of antigen vs MAM plays an important role in determining the effect on the immune response. Furthermore, work is now needed to define the role of MAM on the immune response during active infections with *M. arthritidis*. Studies should also be conducted to determine the role of MAM in *M. arthritidis*-mediated inhibition of the interferon response to viral inducers in vivo (COLE et al. 1975).

6.2 Toxicity and Necrosis

One of the earliest symptoms following the IV injection of large numbers of *M. arthritidis* into mice is the development of a toxic shock syndrome (COLE et al. 1983). Symptoms include lethargy, ruffled fur, conjunctivitis, fecal impaction, and, depending upon dose, death in some individuals. These effects appear due in part to MAM since they were H-2-restricted in that animals whose lymphocytes were MAM-reactive (C3H, B10.D2) were susceptible, whereas mice whose lymphocytes were MAM-nonreactive (C3H.SW, C57BL/10, C3H.B10) were resistant. Susceptible mice also developed extensive peritoneal adhesions after IP injection of organisms. More recent studies using large doses of more highly purified MAM injected IV show a similar toxic syndrome but of much lesser duration and severity. It is likely that the toxic effects of *M. arthritidis* are in part due to the liberation of lymphokines and other inflammatory molecules mediated by MAM-induced activation of lymphocytes and macrophages.

There is evidence that MAM also plays a role in the dermal necrosis induced by *M. arthritidis* after subcutaneous injection of the organisms (COLE et al. 1985a). In this case, mice possessing a functional I-E molecule (C3H, BALB/c, B10.BR, B10.D2) were very susceptible to dermal necrosis, whereas inbred and congenic mice which lacked I-E (C57BL/10, C3H.SW, C3H.B10) developed a suppurative abscess but without dermal damage. In MAM-responsive mice, coagulation type necrosis extended from the suppurative subcutaneous abscess out to the dermis. Few inflammatory cells were seen in this area which was characterized by loss of cellular and nuclear detail, dissolution of the panniculus carnosus muscle, and eventual ulceration. Mice injected with crude unpurified MAM (culture supernatants) failed to show any gross or histological lesions, but studies with pure MAM now need to be undertaken. There is further evidence that MAM may not be entirely responsible for necrosis since a highly virulent strain of *M. arthritidis* can induce some necrosis in I-E-negative mouse strains, and weak necrosis also occurs in BALB/c nu/nu mice. It seems likely, therefore, that MAM renders the host more susceptible to an as yet unidentified necrotizing agent.

6.3 Joint Disease

There are striking differences in *M. arthritidis* disease expression in mice, rats, and rabbits which might relate in part to lymphocyte reactivity to MAM (COLE et al. 1985b). Rabbit lymphocytes fail to respond to MAM and disease in this host can only be obtained by direct injection of organisms into joints. An effective antibody response is produced which rapidly eliminates viable organisms and results in a chronic arthritis mediated by the deposition of immune complexes in cartilage (WASHBURN et al. 1980).

Acute arthritis of mice induced by the systemic injection of virulent *M. arthritidis* is clearly an infectious process. It is not dependent upon MAM since disease develops in many mouse strains irrespective of the responses of their lymphocytes to MAM. Furthermore, MAM does not appear to be associated with virulence of the organisms since nonarthritogenic *M. arthritidis* strains also produce MAM, and high doses of avirulent strains can induce toxicity. It is clear, however, that MAM does have in vivo inflammatory potential, at least in rats (CANNON et al. 1988). Intra-articular injection of DA rats with MAM results in joint swelling characterized by edema below the synovial membrane with polymorphonuclear and focal lymphoid cell infiltration. Subsequently, widespread but incomplete shedding of the synovial membrane, hypertrophy and hyperplasia of the subsynovium with fibroblasts, and the appearance of macrophages occurs. The lesions begin to resolve by day 5 and almost completely disappear by day 7 with healing of the synovial membrane. Repeated exposure of synovial tissues of MAM, as would occur during infection by *M. arthritidis*, might be expected to induce a more chronic phase of arthritis. Of interest is that intra-articular inflammation induced by MAM in BN rats whose lymphocytes are poorly responsive to MAM is much less pronounced.

Most rats recover completely from the acute phase of disease within 6–8 weeks, although a more chronic form of the disease has been described in a small proportion of animals (KIRCHHOFF et al. 1983). After this time, organisms are no longer isolable from the joints and the animals are protected against reinfection. In contrast, mice characteristically develop a more chronic phase of disease. Joint lesions closely resemble those of human RA with massive lymphocytic and plasma cell infiltration of synovium, proliferation of synovial membrane with production of multiple villi, and pannus formation leading to destruction of cartilage and bone (COLE et al. 1971). Of great interest is that the disease can persist for the life of the animal and can exhibit periods of remission and exacerbation which occur commonly in many of the rheumatic diseases. Disease chronicity appears to be associated with continued presence of live organisms, although the latter occur in very small numbers during the chronic stage of disease even in the presence of severe active inflammation. Consistent with the chronicity of the mouse disease is the fact that convalescent sera or cells fail to protect normal mice against disease (COLE et al. 1985b).

Although we do not yet know the role of MAM in the chronic stages of the mouse disease, it is likely to be a major contributor since viable organisms may persist in the joints. It is interesting to speculate that episodes of exacerbation might also be due to multiplication of organisms and MAM production at sites distant from the joints. Since MAM shares some V_β TCR usage with other superantigens, it is possible that infection of mice with other superantigen-producing organisms may also lead to enhanced disease. A further issue to be addressed is whether $V_\beta 6$ or $V_\beta 8$ TCR-bearing T cells play a more direct role in disease by reacting with specific joint components, as is apparently the case with collagen-induced arthritis (HAQQI et al. 1988a, 1988b, 1989) and EAE (HEBER-KATZ and ACHA-ORBEA 1989). Finally, chronic mycoplasma disease in mice may have an autoimmune component since, as we discussed previously, MAM-activated T_H cells can trigger polyclonal B cell proliferation and Ig secretion.

7 Concluding Remarks

MAM has all of the properties characteristic of a superantigen and was, in fact, the first member of this group of proteins to receive detailed study on its requirements for T cell activation. The fact that *M. arthritidis* produces acute systemic disease as well as a chronic relapsing arthritis in rodents led to the proposal that this disease be used as a model system to study the role of superantigens in microbial-mediated chronic diseases (COLE and ATKIN 1991). The availability of numerous mouse strains exhibiting specific mutations or deletions in both the V_β T cell repertoire and in class II MHC antigen expression as well as the growing availability of transgenic mice permits the identification of the specific pathways by which the superantigen, the organism, and the host interact to initiate or perpetuate disease.

The second model system proposed is based upon the use of $V_\beta 6$ and $V_\beta 8$ α/β TCRs by MAM and the association of T cells bearing these same TCRs with type II collagen-induced arthritis of mice (HAQQI et al. 1988a, b). In this model, MAM could be used to determine the role of microbial superantigens in triggering the onset of disease due to preexisting anti-self T cells, to enhancing disease activity by selective clonal expansion of these cells, or to causing an exacerbation of previously resolved disease.

The third model system relates to the ability of MAM to form a superantigen "bridge" between T_H cells and resting B cells, resulting in polyclonal B cell activation (TUMANG et al. 1990). It has been hypothesized that this abnormal T/B cell collaboration could lead to the generation of autoantibodies to repetitive antigen sequences or to multivalent surface antigens as occurs in the antibody-mediated autoimmune diseases such as systemic lupus erythematosus (FRIEDMAN et al. 1991).

Recent studies in our laboratories (B.C. COLE and M.M. GRIFFITHS, unpublished observations) confirm the importance of MAM as a model for superantigen-mediated autoimmune disease. We have demonstrated that systemically-administered MAM can cause a flare of disease activity in mice convalescing from type II collagen-induced arthritis and can also trigger a first episode of arthritis in mice suboptimally immunized with collagen. The respective roles of T cell versus B cell activation in the induction of this autoimmune condition are currently under study.

Further study on the structure of MAM and its interaction with MHC and TCR molecules may also shed light on the Mls self superantigens, which are discussed elsewhere in this volume. The similarity between Mls 1^a and MAM is particularly intriguing since they both use the V$_\beta$6 and V$_\beta$8.1 α/β TCRs and both associate with the I-E molecule for their presentation to the T cell (KAPPLER et al. 1988; MACDONALD et al. 1988; COLE et al. 1990b).

References

Atkin CL, Cole BC, Sullivan GJ, Washburn LR, Wiley BB (1986) Stimulation of mouse lymphocytes by a mitogen derived from *mycoplasma arthritidis*. V. A small basic protein from culture supernatants is a potent T cell mitogen. J Immunol 137: 1581–1589

Bekoff MC, Cole BC, Grey HM (1987) Studies on the mechanism of stimulation of T cells by the *Mycoplasma arthritidis* derived mitogen. Role of class II I-E molecules. J Immunol 139: 3189–3194

Cannon GW, Cole BC, Ward JR (1986) Differential effects of in vitro gold sodium thiomalate on the stimulation of human peripheral mononuclear cells by *Mycoplasma arthritidis* mitogen, concanavalin A, and phytohemagglutinin. J Rheumatol 13: 52–57

Cannon GW, Cole BC, Ward JR, Smith JL, Eichwald EJ (1988) Arthritogenic effects of *Mycoplasma arthritidis* T cell mitogen in rats. J Rheumatol 15: 735–741

Cassell GH, Cole BC (1981) Medical progress: mycoplasmas as agents of human disease. N Engl J Med 304: 80–89

Cole BC (1988) The *Mycoplasma arthritidis* T cell mitogen: a potential new pathway of T cell activation. Clin Immunol Newslett 9: 7–10

Cole BC, Atkin CL (1991) The *Mycoplasma arthritidis* T cell mitogen, MAM: a model superantigen. Immunol Today 12: 271–276

Cole BC, Thorpe RN (1983) Induction of human gamma interferons by a mitogen derived from *Mycoplasma arthritidis* and by phytohemagglutinin: differential inhibition with monoclonal anti-HLA.DR antibodies. J Immunol 131: 2392–2396

Cole BC, Thorpe RN (1984) I-E/I-C region-associated induction of murine gamma interferon by a haplotype-restricted polyclonal T cell mitogen derived from *Mycoplasma arthritidis*. Infect Immune 43: 302–307

Cole BC, Wells DJ (1990) Immunosuppressive properties of the *Mycoplasma arthritidis* T cell mitogen (MAM) in vivo. Infect Immun 58: 228–236

Cole BC, Ward JR, Jones RS, Cahill JF (1971) Chronic proliferative arthritis of mice induced by *Mycoplasma arthritidis*. I. Induction of disease and histopathological characteristics. Infect Immune 4: 344–355

Cole BC, Overall JC Jr, Lombardi PS, Glasgow LA (1975) Mycoplasma-mediated hyporeactivity to various interferon inducers. Infect Immun 12: 1349–1354

Cole BC, Daynes RA, Ward JR (1981) Stimulation of mouse lymphocytes by a mitogen derived from *Mycoplasma arthritidis*. I. Transformation is associated with an H-2-linked gene that maps to the I-E/I-C subregion. J Immunol 127: 1931–1936

Cole BC, Daynes RA, Ward JR (1982a) Stimulation of mouse lymphocytes by a mitogen derived from *Mycoplasma arthritidis*. III. Ir gene control of lymphocyte transformation correlates with binding of the mitogen to specific Ia bearing cells. J Immunol 129: 1352–1359

Cole BC, Sullivan GJ, Daynes RA, Sayed IA, Ward JR (1982b) Stimulation of mouse lymphocytes by a mitogen from *Mycoplasma arthritidis*. II. Cellular requirements for T cell transformation mediated by a soluble mycoplasma mitogen. J Immunol 128: 2013–2018

Cole BC, Washburn LR, Sullivan GJ, Ward JR (1982c) Specificity of a mycoplasma mitogen for lymphocytes from human and various animal hosts. Infect Immun 36: 662–666

Cole BC, Thorpe RN, Hassell LA, Washburn LR, Ward JR (1983) Toxicity but not arthritogenicity of *Mycoplasma arthritidis* for mice associates with the haplotype expressed at the major histocompatibility complex. Infect Immun 41: 1010–1015

Cole BC, Piepkorn MW, Wright EC (1985a) Influence of genes of the major histocompatibility complex on ulcerative dermal necrosis induced in mice by *Mycoplasma arthritidis*. J Invest Dermatol 85: 357–361

Cole BC, Washburn LR, Taylor-Robinson D (1985b) Mycoplasma induced arthritis. In: Razin S, Barile MF (eds) The Mycoplasmas, vol 4. Academic, New York, pp 107–160

Cole BC, Araneo B, Sullivan GJ (1986a) Stimulation of mouse lymphocytes by a mitogen derived from *Mycoplasma arthritidis*. IV. Murine hybridoma cells exhibit differential accessory cell requirements for activation by either *Mycoplasma arthritidis* T cell mitogen, concanavalin A, or hen eggwhite lysozome. J Immunol 136: 3572–3578

Cole BC, Griffiths MM, Sullivan GJ, Ward JR (1986b) Role of non-RT1 genes in the response of rat lymphocytes to *Mycoplasma arthritidis*, T cell mitogen, concanavalin A, and phytohemagglutinin. J Immunol 136: 2364–2369

Cole BC, Kartchner DR, Wells DJ (1989) Stimulation of mouse lymphocytes by a mitogen derived from *Mycoplasma arthritidis*. VII. Responsiveness is associated with expression of a product(s) of the $V_\beta 8$ gene family present on the T cell receptor α/β for antigen. J Immunol 142: 4131–4137

Cole BC, David CS, Lynch DH, Kartchner DR (1990a) The use of transfected fibroblasts and transgenic mice expressing E_a establishes that stimulation of $V_\beta 8$ T cells by the *Mycoplasma arthritidis* mitogen requires E_a. J Immunol 144: 420–424

Cole BC, Kartchner DR, Wells DJ (1990b) Stimulation of mouse lymphocytes by a mitogen derived from *Mycoplasma arthritidis* (MAM). VIII. Selective activation of T cells expressing distinct V_β T cell receptors (TCR) from various strains of mice by the "superantigen" MAM. J Immunol 144: 425–431

Davidson MK, Lindsey JR, Brown MB, Cassell GH, Boorman GA (1983) Natural *Mycoplasma arthritidis* in mice. Curr Microb 8: 205–208

Daynes RA, Novak JM, Cole BC (1982) Comparison of the cellular requirements for human T cell transformation by a soluble mitogen derived from *Mycoplasma arthritidis* and concanavalin A. J Immunol 129: 936–938

Dietz JN, Cole BC (1982) Direct activation of the J774.1 murine macrophage cell line by *Mycoplasma arthritidis*. Infect Immun 37: 811–819

Emery P, Panayi GS, Welsh KI, Cole BC (1985) Rheumatoid factors and HLA- DR4 in rheumatoid arthritis. J Rheumatol 12: 217–222

Fleischer B, Gerardy-Schan R, Metzroth B, Carrel S, Gerlach D, Kohler W (1991) T cell stimulation by microbial toxins: an evolutionary conserved mechanism of T cell activation by microbial toxins. J Immunol 146: 11–17

Friedman SM, Posnett DN, Tumang JR, Cole BC, Crow MK (1991) A potential role for microbial superantigens in the pathogenesis of systemic autoimmune disease. Arthritis Rheum 34: 468–478

Gasser DL, Newlin CM, Palm J, Gonatas NK (1973) Genetic control of susceptibility to experimental allergic encephalomyelitis in rats. Science 181: 872–873

Griffiths MM, DeWitt CW (1984) Modulation of collagen-induced arthritis in rats by non-RT1-linked genes. J Immunol 133: 3043–3046

Haqqi RM, Banerjee S, Behlke MA, Dungeon G, Loh DY, Stuart J, Luthra HS, Davis CS (1988a) $V_\beta 6$ gene of T cell receptor may be involved in type II collagen induced arthritis of mice (Abstr). FASEB J 2: A661

Haqqi RM, Banerjee S, Behlke MA, Dungeon G, Loh DY, Stuart J, Luthra HS, David CS (1988b) Possible role of V_β T cell receptor genes in susceptibility to collagen induced arthritis of mice. J Exp Med 167: 832–839

Haqqi RM, Banerjee S, Anderson GD, David CS (1989) RIIIS/J (H- 2^r): an inbred mouse strain with a massive deletion of T cell receptor V_β genes. J Exp Med 169: 1903–1909

Heber-Katz E, Acha-Orbea H (1989) The V-region disease hypothesis: evidence from autoimmune encephalomyelitis. Immunol Today 10: 164–169

Kappler JW, Staerz U, White J, Marrack PC (1988) T cell receptor, V_β elements which recognize Mls-modified products of the major histocompatibility complex. Nature 332: 35–40

Kirchhoff H, Heitmann J, Ammar A, Hermanns W, Schulz L (1983) Studies of polyarthritis caused by *Mycoplasma arthritidis* in rats. I. Detection of the persisting mycoplasma antigen by the enzyme immune assay (EIA) and conventional culture technique. Zentralbl Bakteriol Mikrobiol Hyg [A] 254: 129–138

Kirchner H, Nicklas W, Giebler D, Keyssner K, Berger R, Storch E (1984) Induction of interferon gamma in mouse spleen cells by culture supernatants of *Mycoplasma arthritidis*. J Interferon Res 4: 389–397

Lynch DH, Cole BC, Bluestone JA, Hodes R (1986) Cross-reactive recognition by antigenspecific, MHC-restricted T cells of a mitogen derived from *Mycoplasma arthritidis* is clonally expressed and I-E restricted. Eur J Immunol 16: 747–751

MacDonald HR, Schneider R, Lees RK, Howe C, Acha-Orbea H, Festenstein H, Zinkernagel RM, Hengartner H (1988) T cell receptor V_β use predicts reactivity and tolerance to Mls^a-encoded antigens. Nature 332: 40–45

Marrack P, Kappler J (1988) The T cell repertoire for antigen and MHC. Immunol Today 9: 308–315

Matthes M, Schrezenmeir H, Homfeld J, Fleischer S, Malissen B, Kirchner H, Fleischer B (1988) Clonal analysis of human T cell activation by the *Mycoplasma arthritidis* mitogen (MAM). Eur J Immunol 18: 1733–1737

Moritz T, Giebler D, Gunther E, Nicklas W, Kirchner H (1984) Lymphoproliferative responses of spleen cells of inbred rats to *Mycoplasma arthritidis* mitogen. Scand J Immunol 20: 365–369

Razin S, Barile MF (1985) The mycoplasmas, vol 4. Mycoplasma pathogenicity. Academic, New York

Stuart PM, Cassell GH, Woodward JG (1990) Differential induction of bone marrow macrophage proliferation by mycoplasmas involves granulocyte-macrophage colony-stimulating factor. Infect Immun 58: 3558–3563

Thirkill CE, Gregerson DS (1982) *Mycoplasma arthritidis*-induced ocular inflammatory disease. Infect Immun 36: 775–781

Tumang JR, Posnet DN, Cole BC, Crow MK, Friedman SM (1990) Helper T cell-dependent human B cell differentiation mediated by a mycoplasmal superantigen bridge. J Exp Med 171: 2153–2158

Ward JR, Jones RS (1962) The pathogenesis of mycoplasmal (PPLO) arthritis in rats. Arthritis Rheum 5: 163–175

Washburn LR, Cole BC, Ward JR (1980) Chronic arthritis of rabbits induced by mycoplasmas. II. Antibody response and the deposition of immune complexes. Arthritis Rheum 23: 837–845

Yowell RL, Cole BC, Daynes RA (1983) Utilization of T cell hybridomas to establish that a soluble factor derived from *Mycoplasma arthritidis* is truly a genetically restricted, polyclonal T cell activator. J Immunol 131: 543–545

The Anti-CD3-Induced Syndrome:
A Consequence of Massive In Vivo Cell Activation

L. Chatenoud, C. Ferran, and J.-F. Bach

1 Introduction

Cytokines constitute an ever growing family of highly potent biological mediators. Our advanced knowledge of the molecular structure of most cytokines, their target receptors, and the respective coding genes contrasts with the still incomplete data available on physiological and pathophysiological regulatory mechanisms operating within the cytokine network. This explains the interest in studying in vivo situations, either in the clinic or in experimental models, where cytokines are directly implicated in the induction of profound sickness or tissue damage. Stimuli described as promoters of monocyte/macrophage or lymphocyte activation, leading to local or systemic cytokine release and pathology, are toxic silicosis (Piguet et al. 1990), bleomycin pneumopathy (Piguet et al. 1989), infectious bacterial endotoxin (Barnett-Sultzer 1968; Skidmore et al. 1975), tuberculosis (Kindler et al. 1989), malaria (Grau et al. 1990), leishmaniosis (Heinzel et al. 1989), or immunological conditions such as graft vs host disease (Piguet et al. 1989b).

More recently, monoclonal antibodies (MoAbs) specifically directed at the CD3 molecule expressed by all mature T lymphocytes (Kung et al. 1979; Clevers et al. 1988) were shown to be, when administered in vivo, very potent inductors of massive systemic cytokine release (Chatenoud et al. 1988, 1989; Abramowicz

---

INSERM U 25, Hôpital Necker, 161 Rue de Sèvres, 75745 Paris, France

et al. 1989; FERRAN et al. 1990a). Importantly, this cytokine release is responsible for an important physical syndrome that constitutes one major side effect in patients receiving anti-CD3 MoAbs for immunosuppression (COSIMI 1987).

The aims of this brief review are to describe the major characteristics of the anti-CD3-induced in vivo activation and to underline its relevance for the study of cytokine-mediated pathological reactions and regulatory circuits.

2 The CD3 Molecule: An Important Target for In Vivo Immunosuppression

OKT3, an anti-human CD3, is the MoAb that has been the most widely used in clinical practice. During initial pilot trials in 1981, the extremely potent and reproducible immunosuppressive capacity of OKT3 became apparent (COSIMI et al. 1981; ORTHO MULTICENTER TRANSPLANT STUDY GROUP 1985). OKT3 was initially selected since, like the polyclonal anti-lymphocyte sera, it is directed to all mature T cells and provokes major T cell lymphopenia, although this is not its exclusive mode of action. Interestingly, it was only after some years, when OKT3 was in frequent use in several transplantation departments for both the treatment and prevention of organ allograft rejection, that the precise molecular structure of its target at the T cell membrane was identified. The CD3 molecule is a complex structure including at least five major polypeptide chains: the γ (25–28 kDa), δ (20 kDa), and ε (20 kDa) chains and the ζ 17 kDa homodimer (BORST et al. 1983, 1984; PESSANO et al. 1985; SAMELSON et al. 1985; CLEVERS et al. 1988). An additional 21 kDa protein linked to some of the CD3 ζ chains has been described in mice (CLEVERS et al. 1988). Tightly linked to the CD3 complex and coprecipitating with it are the two α and β chains of the T cell antigen receptor (TCR) (BORST et al. 1983; MEUER et al. 1983; OETTGEN et al. 1984). All results are concordant in pointing to CD3 as the transduction element of the TCR. This is actually the molecular basis explaining the immunosuppressive potency of OKT3.

Anti-human CD3 MoAbs only cross-react with T cells of some nonhuman primates, namely, chimpanzees and baboons. It was not until recently that a MoAb specific for the murine CD3 molecule was made available. 145-2C11 is a hamster MoAb recognizing the ε chain of the murine CD3 molecule (LEO et al. 1987).

3 Anti-CD3-Induced Acute Syndrome

One very prominent side effect observed in all patients treated with OKT3 is an impressive acute clinical syndrome that follows the first injections of the MoAb. It was originally described as a "flu-like" sickness, associated to a variable degree, depending on the patient, with a large variety of symptoms (COSIMI et al. 1981; COSIMI 1987; GOLDSTEIN et al. 1986). Importantly, the reaction is transient, only observed after the first injections, and spontaneously reversible after 2–3 days of consecutive treatment. The symptoms may be grouped according to three headings based on the severity of the syndrome: (1) Although being a source of major discomfort for the patient, the *high fever*, the *chills*, and the *headache* do not per se have a poor prognosis. (2) The *gastrointestinal symptoms*, i.e., repeated episodes of vomiting and especially diarrhea, are very debilitating since they induce massive fluid and electrolyte loss but can be managed with palliative treatments. (3) The situation is much more complicated in the 10%–15% of patients who experience the more extreme and eventually life threatening symptoms. Among these are the *severe respiratory distress* driven by pulmonary edema, which is observed in patients presenting significant fluid overload at the time of the first OKT3 injection, and the hypotension. It is interesting that hypotension, namely, the shock syndrome, does not represent a regular feature of the OKT3-induced reaction; it is only observed in the small proportion of patients who experience the more severe symptomatology. This element is essential in distinguishing the OKT3-induced reaction from an anaphylactic shock. Indeed, at variance with polyclonal anti-T cell antibodies, despite the thousands of patients treated and even retreated with OKT3, there is no firm documentation of any acute hypersensitivity reaction. The third category of symptoms also includes OKT3-induced neurotoxicity. Some patients may present with nuchal rigidity and confusion: lumbar puncture regularly discloses an aseptic meningitis. A preliminary report suggests that the OKT3-induced neurological toxicity is more frequent when low doses of the MoAb are administered in the absence of any other associated immunosuppressant (RICHARDS et al. 1990). Thus, 54% of patients presenting with solid tumors, in whom a single 50–100 µg i.v. OKT3 injection was injected, showed severe neurotoxicity, as compared to the 10% incidence described in OKT3-treated renal allograft recipients (5 mg/day) (MARTIN et al. 1988).

The OKT3-induced acute reaction is more severe in patients receiving the MoAb for treatment of an ongoing rejection episode than in those treated for prophylaxis. This probably relates to the immune preactivation status of the rejecting patients. The OKT3-induced activation also involves allograft infiltrating T lymphocytes, which explains the transient functional worsening of the rejecting transplant at the beginning of treatment (i.e., transient increase in blood creatinine due to cytokine-promoted vasoactive phenomena).

As in patients, the injection of anti-CD3 into mice induces a major physical reaction. In nongerm-free adult mice, administration of single doses higher than 50–100 µg (2.5–5 mg/kg) are associated with a high mortality (Fig. 1). In totally germ-free adult mice lethality is avoided even at doses as high as 400 µg/mouse (HIRSCH et al. 1988). This indirectly suggests a role for subliminal endotoxin levels (i.e., originating from nonpathogenic digestive tract flora) in potentiating the cytokine-induced syndrome. Using lower doses (5–20 µg/mouse) animals are sick but, as in patients, the syndrome spontaneously reverses after 48–72 h. Mice experience prostration and hypomotility (that may be quantitated using an

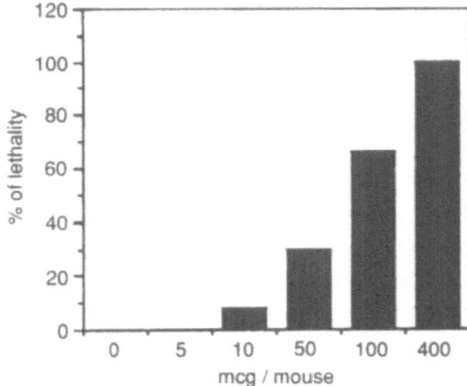

Fig. 1. Lethality in 145-2C11 treated mice

actimetric device), hypothermia (the equivalent of fever in humans since rodents are not homeotherms), diarrhea, and piloerection.

4 Anti-CD3-Induced Cytokine Release

From a biological point of view, the anti-CD3-induced syndrome is the in vivo counterpart of the in vitro mitogenic properties of the MoAb.

All anti-CD3 MoAbs so far described have a potent T cell mitogenic activity extensively studied. This activity is monocyte-dependent, since F(ab)'2 are not mitogenic (VAN WAUVE et al. 1980; CHANG et al. 1981), and significantly varies depending on the isotype of the murine antibody (IgG2a ≫ IgG1 ≫ IgG2b) (VAN LIER et al. 1987). This parallels the variable affinity of human monocyte Fc receptors for murine IgG isotypes, shown to be HLA-related. The in vitro proliferative response is of course associated with significant cytokine release (CUTURI et al. 1987).

These results were a logical starting point to hypothesize that transient cell activation leading to cytokine release was the cause of the anti-CD3 syndrome. In addition, since all the symptoms elicited were quite reminiscent of those reported in patients receiving exogenous recombinant cytokines (REMICK et al. 1987; ROSENBERG et al. 1987). In humans this could directly be demonstrated when specific radioimmunoassays for cytokine dosage were made available, that offered enormous technical advantages over the conventional bioassays.

In all patients, as early as 1 h after the first OKT3 injection, massive release of tumor necrosis factor (TNF) is observed in the circulation. In some patients, values are definitely higher (around 2000 pg/ml) than the ones detected in septic shock. In contrast to TNF release, in no case could any interleukin (IL)-1β be detected. At 4 h after the injection, exclusively T cell-derived cytokines such as interferon-γ (IFN-γ) and IL-2 also peak in the circulation (CHATENOUD et al. 1988, 1989; ABRAMOWICZ et al. 1989). IL-6 is also released 3–6 h after the injection. Although massive, this cytokine release is self-limited. It exclusively follows the first OKT3 injection and all cytokines return to pretreatment levels by 20 h postinjection, except IL-6 which may show a longer lasting kinetics (36–48 h after the first injection).

Fully comparable results were obtained in anti-CD3-treated mice (FERRAN et al. 1990a; ALEGRE et al. 1990). Significant levels of TNF, IFN-γ, IL-2, IL-3, and IL-6 could be detected in the serum of BALB/c mice injected with 10 µg of anti-CD3 (FERRAN et al. 1990a). By 24 h after the injection, significant anatomo pathological lesions are evidenced that involve lymphoid organs and tissues known to be the main targets of the released cytokines, namely, the lung and the liver. A pneumonia-like picture, including inflammatory cell infiltration, diffuse vascular congestion, and even thrombosis, is observed in the lungs of treated mice; cell vacuolization, cell necrosis and vascular congestion is the rule in the liver (FERRAN et al. 1990a). The pattern of cytokines released clearly pointed to the cellular elements most actively involved in the reaction. In fact, although anti-CD3 MoAbs induce in vivo T cell opsonization and subsequent lysis, an exclusive activation of reticuloendothelial cells through these mechanisms could be ruled out. First, other anti-T cell MoAbs, including anti-CD2, anti-CD4, or anti-CD8, although inducing T cell opsonization with more or less pronounced lympholysis both in experimental models (monkeys, rats, or mice) (JONKER et al. 1983; BENJAMIN et al. 1986) and in humans (HAFLER et al. 1988; GOLDBERG et al., submitted), do not provoke massive cytokine release. Second, in case of exclusive activation of monocytes/macrophages, as described following injection of Escherichia coli endotoxin into either normal volunteers or mice, only TNF is detected in the circulation (MICHIE et al. 1988). Similarly, passive release of cytokines from lysed cells is improbable since it is well-known that the amount of biologically active cytokines stored within cells is negligible.

Thus, all results are concordant in suggesting that T lymphocytes are the major source for most, if not all, the cytokines produced. Even in the case of TNF, our preliminary data on purified spleen cell populations suggest that activated T splenocytes, recovered from anti-CD3-treated mice, are TNF producers. It is worth mentioning at this point that the transient lymphocyte activation is also well-evidenced, both in humans and mice, by the expression of functional IL-2 receptors at the surface of T cells located in profound lymphoid organs (HIRSCH et al. 1989; ELLENHORN et al. 1990). Following the first anti-CD3 injection, cell depletion is complete in the periphery but only partial within lymphoid organs; remnant T cells undergo antigenic modulation of the CD3/TCR complex (CHATENOUD and BACH 1984).

Nevertheless, all these arguments do not preclude the active participation of monocytes/macrophages in the reaction. Data from mice are clear-cut in confirming the nonactivating property of anti-CD3 F(ab')2 fragments. Just as they do in vitro, F(ab')2 fragments injected in vivo, even at very high doses (100–200 µg/mouse), do not elicit either the cytokine release or the physical syndrome (HIRSCH et al. 1990; CHATENOUD et al., submitted).

The importance of the epitope recognized on the CD3/TCR complex in determining such a massive T cell activation is well-illustrated by the example of a MoAb specific for the constant portion of human TCR (BMA 031). In vitro, BMA 031 is less mitogenic than OKT3. When injected in vivo BMA 031 is very well-tolerated despite the fact it induces, like OKT3, TNF release. However, in contrast to OKT3, no other cytokine is detected (CHATENOUD et al., submitted). These data suggest that TNF alone is insufficient in giving rise to the clinical syndrome.

5 Variabilities in Anti-CD3-Induced Activation Among Murine Strains

By analogy with studies performed on lipopolysaccharide (LPS), we undertook a comparison analysis of the anti-CD3-induced activation among four murine strains. The idea was first to define variable patterns of anti-CD3-induced cytokine release in different inbred mice populations that could then allow to better define the precise role of each cytokine released in mediating the physical syndrome. BALB/c and CBA/J are good responders to LPS, produce high levels of colony-stimulating factor (CSF) and TNF after LPS injection, and exhibit a severe physical reaction that is lethal at high LPS doses (BARNETT-SULTZER 1968; SKIDMORE et al. 1975). NZW mice express an abnormal restriction fragment length polymorphism of the TNF gene correlated with reduced in vitro TNF production by peritoneal macrophages following LPS and IFN-γ stimulation (JACOB and MCDEVITT 1988). C3H/HeJ mice represent the reference LPS "resistant" strain. C3H/HeJ mice exhibit a dual defect in both TNF mRNA transcription and protein production is response to LPS related to a single mutation involving the *Mup* 1 or *lps* d (defective) gene on the fourth chromosome (WATSON et al. 1978; BEUTLER et al. 1986a).

Following anti-CD3 injection, a quite different pattern of both disease and cytokine release was observed among the four strains. BALB/c mice experienced the most severe reaction with profound hypothermia (Table 1), hypomotility, and a 100% incidence of diarrhea. Anti-CD3-treated CBA/J mice showed a less severe reaction than BALB/c with only moderate hypothermia, hypomotility, and less frequent diarrhea (40% of the animals). However, in this strain the reaction lasted longer; total reversal occurred at 72 h as compared to 48 h in the three other strains. NZW mice showed mild hypothermia and hypomotility. Finally, C3H/HeJ mice were almost not affected, showing modest hypomotility as the only symptom.

Table 1. Body temperature in different mice strains following 145 2C11 treatment

Mice strain		145 2C11 Treatment			
		Before injection	4 h after injection	24 h after injection	48 h after injection
BALB/c	Treated	38.2 ± 0.06	34.4 ± 0.32	34.6 ± 0.15	37.1 ± 0.12
	Controls	38.3 ± 0.05 (NS)	38.2 ± 0.06 ($p < 0.0001$)	37.2 ± 0.19 ($p < 0.0001$)	37.9 ± 0.15 ($p = 0.002$)
NZW	Treated	38.5 ± 0.09	36.9 ± 0.12	37.2 ± 0.10	37.4 ± 0.21
	Controls	38.2 ± 0.25 (NS)	38.01 ± 0.10 ($p < 0.0001$)	37.3 + 0.17 (NS)	37.6 ± 0.22 (NS)
CBA/J	Treated	38.4 ± 0.10	36.3 ± 0.15	37.5 ± 0.21	37.3 ± 0.18
	Controls	38.4 ± 0.09 (NS)	37.7 ± 0.19 ($p < 0.0001$)	37.5 ± 0.19 (NS)	37.5 ± 0.18 (NS)
C3H/HeJ	Treated	38.1 ± 0.16	37.1 ± 0.14	38.3 ± 0.14	37.1 ± 0.15
	Controls	37.8 ± 0.19 (NS)	36.8 ± 0.17 (NS)	37.2 ± 0.21 (NS)	37.1 ± 0.22 (NS)

Body temperature is expressed in °C. Results refer to mean ± SEM values obtained from 4–6 different experiments for each mouse strain analyzed

Table 2. Serum TNF levels in 145-2C11 treated mice strains

Time	BALB/c	CBA/J	C3H/HeJ	NZW
1 h after injection	64 ± 9.8	52 ± 12	96 ± 6	144 ± 46
4 h after injection	0	0	0	12 ± 4.9

TNF L929 bioassay levels are expressed in units/ml (mean ± SEM)

All this correlated with significant variations in the pattern of cytokines released. TNF was present in all four strains (Table 2). Peak levels were observed 90 min after anti-CD3 injection. No correlation could be evidenced between TNF levels and the severity of the physical reaction. Indeed, BALB/c, which was the most affected strain, presented TNF circulating levels not different from those scored in the other three strains. One must underline that in NZW and LPS resistant C3H/HeJ mice a normal pattern of anti-CD3-induced TNF was found. Since C3H/HeJ monocytes/macrophages were reported not to produce TNF (WATSON et al. 1978; BEUTLER et al. 1986a), one may question whether the protein detected after anti-CD3 in these mice is T cell-derived or alternatively, is triggered by another activation pathway (Fc receptor-related), different from the one stimulated by LPS. A third possibility is that either anti-CD3 itself or the other cytokines released can overcome the C3H/HeJ resistance. Some data suggested that IFN-γ mediate this effect in C3H/HeJ mice (BEUTLER et al. 1986b).

Table 3. Serum IFN-γ levels in BALB/c mice after 145-2C11 treatment

Time	IFN-γ level (units/ml)
Before 145-2C11	0
Before 145-2C11	0
90 min after the injection	7 ± 2
4 h after the injection	10 ± 3.13
8 h after the injection	3 ± 3

BALB/c mice were unique in presenting significant serum IFN-γ levels 4–8 h after anti-CD3 injection (Table 3). Thus, the anti-CD3-induced physical reaction seems more severe when both TNF and IFN-γ are present. This observation is in keeping with the well-described synergism between these two cytokines (PHILIP and EPSTEIN 1986; TALMADGE et al. 1987), at least partly due to up-modulation of TNF receptors by IFN-γ (AGGARWAL et al. 1985; TSUJIMOTO et al. 1986).

In all four strains, IL-3 was present 4–8 h after anti-CD3 injection. The highest levels were noted in the most severely affected animals, namely, in BALB/c and CBA/J mice. Moreover, in CBA/J mice, IL-3 was still detectable 24 h after anti-CD3 injection in association with granulocyte/macrophage colony-stimulating factor (GM-CSF). This suggests a role of IL-3/GM-CSF in the long-lasting hypomotility noted in this strain.

Based on these results TNF seems to play a key role in the pathophysiology of the anti-CD3-induced reaction, although it is evident that synergy with other cytokines, mainly IFN-γ, IL-3/GM-CSF, and probably also IL-6, is mandatory for eliciting the typical physical syndrome. These conclusions led to the experiments using anti-TNF MoAbs in the prevention of the anti-CD3-induced reaction. As we shall describe below, such a strategy fully confirmed that TNF is an essential link in the cytokine cascade elicited by anti-CD3.

No difference was noted among the tested strains in serum IL-2 levels. However, one cannot exclude at this point its responsibility in potentiating some of the anti-CD3 side effects either directly or again via synergy with other cytokines.

6 Modulation of Anti-CD3-Induced Cytokine Release

Several means can be envisaged to modulate anti-CD3-induced activation. However, we shall concentrate on two types of strategies, which have both fundamental and clinical relevance.

6.1 Modulation by Corticosteroids

Corticosteroids are potent inhibitors of both endotoxin-induced cytokine release and mortality (ZUCKERMAN et al. 1989). Similarly, in OKT3-treated human allograft recipients, the intensity of the acute clinical syndrome and the serum levels of induced cytokines are significantly reduced when high dose corticosteroids (7–10 mg/kg of methylprednisolone as a single i.v. bolus) are given before the first MoAb injection (CHATENOUD et al. 1990). This provides the rationale for using this therapeutic procedure, initially applied on an empirical basis, since it was the only available means to decrease the severity of at least some of the OKT3-induced acute symptoms. The variability in results presented by different centers is due to differences in the corticosteroid administration protocols (dosages but mostly scheduling (ABRAMOWICZ et al. 1989; CHATENOUD et al. 1990).

We took advantage of the murine model to define the optimal protocol. Mice were pretreated with 1 mg sodium hydrocortisone succinate 1,4 or 12 h prior to anti-CD3 injection (FERRAN et al. 1990b). Results showed that only when administered 1 h prior to anti-CD3 injection, were high dose corticosteroids able to significantly decrease cytokine production, leading to a beneficial effect on at least some of the anti-CD3-related physical symptoms. Adequate corticosteroid pretreatment completely reversed the hypothermia at 4 h postinjection and modestly affected the diarrhea (seen in 50% of the animals as compared to 100% controls). By contrast, hypomotility was almost unaffected by corticosteroids. Nonetheless, the beneficial effect was transient, occurring at 4 h following anti-CD3 administration but disappearing later on.

Anti-CD3-induced cytokine release was also affected by corticosteroid pretreatment. Results showed an 85% decrease in circulating IL-2 levels; IFN-γ and IL-6 serum levels were significantly reduced 90 min after anti-CD3 injection but at 4 h the levels were comparable to those detected in controls (animals receiving anti-CD3 without corticosteroid pretreatment). In the case of anti-CD3-induced TNF, corticosteroids promoted a significant decrease at 90 min followed by a clear-cut rebound at 4 h (FERRAN et al. 1990b).

Corticosteroids affect cytokine production in various ways. They may inhibit specific messenger RNA transcription or act at a posttranscriptional level, thus repressing protein synthesis (as is the case for TNF, IL-6, and IFN-γ) (ARYA et al. 1984; REED et al. 1986; LEE et al. 1988).

To confirm the clinical validity of these results, a small, randomized, prospective trial, including 12 consecutive patients receiving high dose corticosteroids (0.5 g/methylprednisolone) either before or at the time of the first OKT3 injection, was performed (CHATENOUD et al. 1991). Results confirmed that corticosteroids must be given 1 h before the first OKT3 injection to significantly decrease TNF and IFN-γ release. In addition, as in mice, pretreatment with corticosteroids totally abolished the OKT3-induced IL-2 release. These results provide a biological basis for a precise administration schedule of high dose corticosteroids in order to exert the best inhibition of anti-CD3-induced cytokine production.

6.2 Modulation by Anti-Cytokine Antibodies

The purpose of evaluating the effects of anti-TNF and anti-IFN-γ on the anti-CD3 reaction was dual: first, to better define the respective role of TNF and IFN-γ in the cytokine cascade, and second, to find a therapeutic strategy applicable to patients that could abrogate the anti-CD3 syndrome.

The antibodies used were: the hamster anti-murine TNF MoAb TN3-19.12 and the hamster anti-murine IFN-γ MoAb H-22 (kindly provided by R. Schreiber and K. Sheehan). A polyclonal anti-murine TNF (kindly provided by G. Grau and P. Vassalli) was also tested n parallel. All these antibodies were shown to block in vitro and in vivo the bioactivity of the respective cytokine.

BALB/c mice were pretreated with an adequate dose of each antibody alone or in combination with anti-TNF and anti-IFN-γ MoAbs before receiving anti-CD3. Mice pretreated with anti-TNF significantly improved as compared to control animals (pretreated with a control hamster MoAb). In these animals, hypothermia was completely reversed, diarrhea was absent (as compared to a 100% incidence in controls), and hypomotility was significantly improved. Mice pretreated with the polyclonal anti-TNF antibody also showed a noticeable benefit. In contrast, mice pretreated with anti-IFN-γ MoAbs did not show any improvement in the physical reaction.

Animals pretreated with the combination of anti-TNF and anti-IFN-γ MoAbs showed less improvement than animals given anti-TNF antibodies alone, only evidenced at 4 h after anti-CD3 injections. Further on, anti-TNF + anti-IFN-γ pretreated mice were as sick as control animals (FERRAN et al. 1991).

Detailed analysis of the levels and kinetics of cytokine release provided further insights into the mode of action in this model of the anti-cytokine MoAbs. Results suggested that blockable of TNF biological activity was not the only mechanism explaining the beneficial effect of the anti-TNF MoAb on the anti-CD3-induced reaction. Anti-TNF administration totally modified the pattern of most of the other released cytokines (Tables 4 and 5). Experiments were concordant in showing a significant increase in circulating anti-CD3-induced IFN-γ levels in anti-TNF-pretreated animals. The increase was evident at the peak time point, namely, 4 h after anti-CD3 injection, and was still detectable at 8 h (Table 4). The augmented IFN-γ levels correlated with a significant and reproducible decrease in both anti-CD3-induced IL-3 and IL-6 levels (Table 5). Conversely, in anti-IFN-γ pretreated animals, circulating TNF levels were identical to controls and total blockade of circulating IFN-γ bioactivity was observed associated with a significant increase in circulating IL-3 and IL-6 levels (Table 5).

These data strongly suggest that the beneficial effect of anti-TNF MoAbs on the anti-CD3-induced reaction seems to be associated with the up-regulation of IFN-γ levels, which in turn contribute, to the IL-3 and IL-6 decrease (FERRAN et al. 1991). This is further stressed by results indicating that anti-IFN-γ may abrogate the beneficial effect of anti-TNF MoAb pretreatment.

Finally, one may add that anti-CD3-induced IL-2 was not modified by either anti-TNF or anti-IFN-γ MoAb pretreatment. Once T cell activation occurred, IL-2

Table 4. IFN-γ levels in mice receiving either anti-TNF MoAb or the L2 control MoAb prior to 145 2C11

Time	Anti-TNF + anti-CD3 (U/ml)	L2 + anti-CD3 (U/ml)
0	0	0
90 min	4 ± 4	7 ± 2
4 h	40 ± 11	10 ± 3.6
8 h	16 ± 4	0

Table 5. Serum IL-3 and IL-6 levels at various times (T) in mice pretreated with anti-TNF and or anti-IFN-γ Moabs prior to 145-2C11 injection

Time	Anti-TNF/anti-CD3 (U/ml)	Anti-IFNγ/anti-CD3 (U/ml)	Anti-TNF + anti-IFNγ/anti-CD3 (U/ml)	L2/anti-CD3 (U/ml)
IL-6 LEVELS				
T-0	16.3 ± 4.63	17 ± 7	24.4 ± 13.5	19.5 ± 10.5
T-90 min	1524 ± 10	10940 ± 2575	667 ± 100	3295 ± 673
T-4 h	4732 ± 100	5680 ± 448	2025 ± 1039	3479 ± 42
T-8 h	779 ± 176	2809 ± 549	701 ± 217	5501 ± 171
T-24 h	385 ± 31	1196 ± 158	408 ± 58	344 ± 106
Histamine-producing cell stimulating activity (HCSA) Levels				
T-0	0	7 ± 2	4.5 ± 3.5	0
T-4 h	123 ± 18	754 ± 135	237 ± 23	323 ± 74
T-8 h	84 ± 21.5	536 ± 90	195 ± 60	271 ± 15
T-24 h	7 ± 3.4	118 ± 26	41.5 ± 0.7	4U ± 1

production seemed less susceptible to regulation by other cytokines. Conversely, as previously mentioned, IL-2 is the anti-CD3-induced cytokine whose levels are the most affected by pretreatment with high doses of corticosteroids.

These results could be reproduced in OKT3-treated patients. A pilot clinical trial was set up, including OKT3-treated renal allograft recipients who received an anti-human TNF MoAb 1 h prior to the first MoAb injection. This pretreatment almost completely abrogated the OKT3 syndrome.

7 Conclusion

Anti-CD3 MoAbs represent a stimuli that elicit in vivo a masssive monocyte-dependent T cell activation and cytokine release. These antibodies trigger a major physiological activation pathway of T lymphocytes through the

CD3/TCR molecule. The murine model using the 145-2C11 MoAb represents valuable tool to approach practical issues related to the clinical use of anti-CD3 antibodies. It allows to test the effectiveness of therapeutic strategies aimed at preventing the anti-CD3-induced syndrome. In addition, provided major insights into the physiology of the cytokine cascade and the synergisms between these soluble mediators that are essential in provoking the anti-CD3-mediated syndrome. Results are concordant in suggesting a pivotal role for TNF and TNF-mediated modulation of IFN-γ in the anti-CD3-induced syndrome. From a fundamental point of view, it is essential to determine whether TNF-mediated IFN-γ regulation is a pretranscriptional event or relies on a modification of cytokine consumption via modulation of receptor expression.

Interfering with the cytokine cascade triggered by anti-CD3 using anti-TNF MoAbs was highly effective in preventing one major side effect linked to in vivo use of anti-CD3 MoAbs.

References

Abramowicz D, Schandenne L, Goldman M, Crusiaux A, Vereerstraeten P, de Pauw L, Wybran J, Kinnaert P, Dupont E, Toussaint C (1989) Release of tumor necrosis factor, interleukin 2, and gamma-interferon in serum after injection of OKT3 monoclonal antibody in kidney transplant recipients. Transplantation 47: 606–613

Aggarwal BB, Eessalu TE, Hass PE (1985) Characterization of receptors for human tumor necrosis factor and their regulation by γ interferon. Nature 318: 665–667

Apte RN, Pluznik DH (1976) Genetic control of lipopolysaccharide induced generation of serum colony stimulating factor and proliferation of splenic granulocyte/macrophage precursor cells. J Cell Physiol 89: 313–323

Alegre M, Vandenabeele P, Flamand V, Moser M, Leo O, Abramowicz D, Urbain J, Fiers W, Goldman M (1990) Hypothemia and hypoglycemia induced by anti-CD3 monoclonal antibody in mice; role of tumor necrosis factor. Eur J Immunol 20: 707–710

Arya SK, Wong-Staal F, Gallo RC (1984) Dexamethasone-mediated inhibition of human T cell growth factor and γ-interferon messenger RNA. J Immunol 133: 273–276

Barnett-Sultzer (1968) Genetic control of leucocyte responses to endotoxin. Nature 219: 1253–1254

Benjamin RJ, Cobbod SP, Clark MR, Waldmann H (1986) Tolerance to rat monoclonal antibodies. J Exp Med 163: 1539–1552

Beutler B, Krochin N, Milsark IW, Luedke C, Cerami A (1986a) Control of cachectin (tumor necrosis factor) synthesis: mechanisms of endotoxin resistance. Science 232: 977–980

Beutler B, Tkacenko V, Milsark I, Krochin N, Cerami A (1986b) Effect of γ interferon on cachectin expression by mononuclear phagocytes. Reversal of the (lps d) (endoxin resistance) phenotype. J Exp Med 164: 1791–1796

Borst J, Alexander S, Elder J, Terhorst C (1983) The T3 complex on human T lymphocytes involves four structurally distinct glycoproteins. J Biol Chem 258: 5135–5141

Borst J, Colligan JE, Oettgen H, Pessano S, Malin R, Terhorst C (1984) The gamma and epsilon chains of the human T3/T cell receptor complex are distinct polypeptides. Nature 312: 455–458

Chang TW, Kung PC, Gingras SP, Goldstein G (1981) Does OKT3 monoclonal antibody react with an antigen-recognition structure on human T cells? Proc Natl Acad Sci USA 78: 1805–1808

Chatenoud L, Bach JF (1984) Antigenic modulation. A major mechanism of antibody action. Immunol Today 5: 20–25

Chatenoud L, Ferran C, Reuter A, Franchimont P, Legendre C, Kreis H, Bach JF (1988) Clinical use of OKT3: the role of cytokine release and xenosensitization. J Autoimmun 1: 631–639

Chatenoud L, Ferran C, Reuter A, Legendre C, Gevaert Y, Kreis H, Franchimont P, Bach JF (1989) Systemic reaction to the monoclonal antibody OKT3 in relation to serum levels of tumor necrosis factor and interferon γ. N Engl J Med 320: 1420–1421

Chatenoud L, Ferran C, Legendre C, Thouard I, Merite S, Reuter A, Gevaert Y, Kreis H, Franchimont P, Bach JF (1990) In vivo cell activation following OKT3 administration; systemic cytokine release and modulation by corticosteroids. Transplantation 49: 697–702

Chatenoud L, Legendre C, Ferran C, Bach JF, Kreis H (1991) Corticosteroids inhibition of the OKT3 induced cytokine related syndrome-dosage and kinetics prerequisites. Transplantation 51 (in press)

Clevers H, Alarcon B, Wileman T, Terhorst C (1988) The T cell receptor/CD3 complex: dynamic protein ensemble. Annu Rev Immunol 6: 629–662

Cosimi AB (1987) Clinical development of orthoclone OKT3. Transplant Proc [Suppl 1] 14: 7–16

Cosimi AB, Colvin RB, Burton RC, Rubin RH, Goldstein G, Kung PC, Hansen P, Delmonico FL, Russel PS (1981) Use of monoclonal antibodies to T-cell subsets for immunologic monitoring and treatment in recipients of renal allografts. N Engl J Med 305: 308–314

Cuturi MC, Murphy M, Costa-Giomi MP, Weinmann R, Perussia B, Trinchieri G (1987) Independant regulation of tumor necrosis factor and lymphotoxin production by human peripheral blood lymphocytes. J Exp Med 165: 1581–1584

Ellenhorn JDI, Woodle ES, Ghobreal I, Thistlethwaite JR, Bluestone J (1990) Activation of human T cells in vivo following treatment of transplant recipients with OKT3. Transplantation 50: 608–612

Ferran C, Sheehan C, Dy M, Schreiber R, Merite S, Landais P, Noel LH, Grau G, Bluestone J, Bach JF, Chatenoud L (1990a) Cytokine related syndrome following injection of anti-CD3 monoclonal antibody: further evidence for transient in vivo T cell activation. Eur J Immunol 20: 509–515

Ferran C, Dy M, Merite S, Sheehan K, Schreiber R, Leboulenger F, Landais P, Bluestone JA, Bach JF, Chatenoud L (1990b) Corticosteroids reduce morbidity and cytokine release in anti-CD3 MoAb treated mice. Transplantation 50: 642–648

Ferran C, Sheehan K, Schreiber R, Bach JF, Chatenoud L (1991) Anti-TNF abrogates the cytokine related anti-CD3 induced syndrome. Transplant Proc 23(1): 849–850

Goldstein G, Norman DJ, Shield CF, Kreis H, Burdick J (1986) OKT3 monoclonal antibody reversal of acute renal allograft rejection unresponsive to conventional immunosuppressive treatments. In: (Meryman HT (ed)) Transplantation: approaches to graft rejection. Liss, New York, pp 239–249

Grau G, Frei K, Piguet PF, Fontana A, Heremans H, Billiau A, Vassalli P, Lambert PH (1990) Interleukin 6 production in experimental cerebral malaria: modulation by anticytokine antibodies and possible role of hypergammaglobulinemia. J Exp Med 172: 1505–1508

Hafler DA, Ritz J, Schlossmann SF, Weiner HL (1988) Anti-CD4 and anti-CD2 monoclonal antibody infusions in subjects with multiple sclerosis. Immunosuppressive effect and anti-mouse immune response. J Immunol 141: 131–138

Heinzel FP, Sadick MP, Holaday BJ, Coffman RL, Locksley RM (1989) Reciprocal expression of interferon γ or interleukin 4 during the resolution or progression of murine leishmaniasis. J Exp Med 169: 59–72

Hirsch R, Eckhaus M, Auchincloss H Jr, Sachs DH, Bluestone JA (1988) Effects of in vivo administration of anti-T3 monoclonal antibody on T cell function in mice. I. Immunosuppression of transplantation responses. J Immunol 140: 3766–3772

Hirsch R, Gress RE, Pluznik DH, Eckhaus M, Bluestone JA (1989) Effects of in vivo administration of anti-T3 monoclonal antibody on T cell function in mice. II. In vivo activation of T cells. J Immunol 142: 737–743

Hirsch R, Bluestone JA, DeNenno L, Gress RE (1990) Anti-CD3 F(ab')2 fragments are immunosuppressive in vivo without evoking either the strong humoral response or morbidity associated with whole mAb. Transplantation 49: 1117–1123

Jacob CO, McDevitt HO (1988) Tumour necrosis factor-α in murine autoimmune "lupus" nephritis. Nature 331: 356–358

Jonker M, Goldstein G, Balner H (1983) Effects of in vivo administration of monoclonal antibodies specific for human T cell subpopulations on the immune system in a Rhesus monkey model. Transplantation 35: 521–526

Kindler V, Sappino AP, Grau GE, Piguet PF, Vassali P (1989) The inducing role of tumor necrosis factor in the development of bactericidal granulomas during BCG infection. Cell 56: 731–740

Kung PC, Goldstein G, Reinherz E, Schlossman SF (1979) Monoclonal antibodies defining distinctive human T-cell surface antigens. Science 206: 347–349

Lee SW, Tsou AP, Chan H (1988) Dexamethasone mediated inhibition of human T cell growth factor and γ-interferon messenger RNA. Proc Natl Acad Sci USA 85: 1204–1208

Leo O, Foo M, Sachs DH, Samelson LE, Buestone SA (1987) Identification of a monoclonal antibody specific for a murine T3 polypeptide. Proc Natl Acad Sci (USA) 84: 1374–1377

Martin MA, Massanari RM, Nghiem DD, Smith JL, Corry RJ (1988) Nosocomial aseptic meningitis associated with administration of OKT3. JAMA 259: 2002–2005

Meuer SC, Fitzgerald KA, Hussey RE, Hodgdon JC, Schlossman SF, Reinherz EL (1983) Clonotypic structures involved in antigen specific human T cell function. Relationship to the T3 molecular complex. J Exp Med 157: 705–719

Michie HR, Manogue KR, Sprigs DR, Revhaug A, O'Dwyer S, Dinarello CA, Cerami A, Wolff SM, Wilmore DW (1988) Detection of circulating tumor necrosis factor after endotoxin administration. N Engl J Med 318: 1481–1486

Oettgen H, Kappler J, Tax WJM, Terhorst C (1984) Characterization of the two heavy chains of the T3 complex on the surface of human T lymphocytes. J Biol Chem 259: 12039–12048

Ortho Multicenter Transplant Study Group (1985) A randomized clinical trial of OKT3 monoclonal antibody for acute rejection of cadaveric renal transplants. N Engl J Med 313: 337–342

Pessano S, Oettgen H, Bhan AK, Terhorst C (1985) The T3/T cell receptor complex: antigenic distinction between the 20 kDa T3 (T3-δ and T3-δ) subunits. EMBO J 4: 337–344

Philip R, Epstein LB (1986) Tumour necrosis factor as immunomodulator and mediator of monocyte cytotoxicity induced by itself, γ interferon and interleukin-1. Nature 323: 86–89

Piguet PF, Grau G, Collart MA, Vassalli P, Kapanci Y (1989) Pneumopathies of the graft versus host reaction. Lab Invest 61: 37–45

Piguet PF, Collart MA, Grau G, Sappino AP, Vassalli P (1990) Requirement of tumor necrosis factor for development of the silica-induced pulmonary fibrosis. Nature 344: 245–247

Reed JC, Abidi AH, Alpers JD, Hoover RG, Robb RJ, Nowell PC (1986) Effect of cyclosporin A and dexamethasone on interleukin 2 receptor gene expression. J Immunol 137: 150–154

Remick DG, Kungel RG, Larrick JW, Kunkel SL (1987) Acute in vivo effects of human recombinant tumor necrosis factor. Lab Invest 56: 583–590

Richards JM, Vogelzang NJ, Bluestone JA (1990) Neurotoxicity after treatment with muromonab-CD3. N Engl J Med 323: 487

Rosenberg SA, Lotze MT, Mutt LM, Chang AE, Avis FP, Leitman S, Linehan N, Robertson CN, Lee RE, Rubin JT, Seipp CA, Simpson CG, White DE (1987) A progress report on the treatment of 157 patients with advanced cancer using lymphokine-activated killer cells and interleukin-2 or high dose interleukin-2 alone. N Engl J Med 316: 889–897

Samelson LE, Harford JB, Klausner RD (1985) Identification of the components of the murine T cell antigen receptor complex. Cell 43: 223–231

Schreiber RD, Hicks LJ, Celada A, Buchmeier NA, Gray PW (1985) Monoclonal antibodies to murine γ-interferon which differentially modulate macrophage activation and anti-viral activity. J Immunol 134: 1609–1618

Sheehan KCF, Ruddle NH, Schreiber RD (1989) Generation and characterization of hamster monoclonal antibodies that neutralize murine tumor necrosis factors. J Immunol 142: 3884–3893

Skidmore BJ, Chiller JC, Morrison DC, Weigle WO (1975) Immunologic properties of bacterial lipopolysaccharide (LPS): correlation between the mitogenic, adjuvant, and immunogenic activities. J Immunol 114: 770–778

Sultzer BM (1968) Genetic control of leucocyte response to endotoxin. Nature 219: 1253–1254

Talmadge JE, Bowersox O, Tribble H, Lee SH, Shepard HM, Liggitt D (1987) Toxicity of tumor necrosis factor is synergistic with γ interferon and can be reduced with cyclooxygenase inhibitors. Am J Pathol 128: 410–425

Tsujimoto M, Yip YK, Vilcek J (1986) Interferon γ enhances expression of cellular receptors for tumor necrosis factor. J Immunol 136: 2441–2450

Van Lier RAW, Boot JHA, de Groot ER, Aarden LA (1987) Induction of T cell proliferation with anti-CD3 switch-variant monoclonal antibodies; effects of heavy chain isotype in monocyte dependent systems. Eur J Immunol 17: 1599–1604

Van Wauwe JP, de May JR, Goossens JG (1980) OKT3: a monoclonal anti-human T lymphocyte antibody with potent mitogenic properties. J Immunol 124: 2708–2713

Watson J, Largen M, McAdam KPWJ (1978) Genetic control of endotoxin responses in mice. J Exp Med 147: 39–49

Wofsy D, Seaman WE (1985) Successful treatment of autoimmunity in NZB/NZW F$_1$ mice with monoclonal antibody to L3T4. J Exp Med 161: 378–391

Zuckerman SH, Shellhaas J, Butler LD (1989) Differential regulation of lipopolysaccharide-induced interleukin 1 and tumor necrosis factor synthesis: effects of endogenous and exogenous glucocorticoids and the role of the pituitary-adrenal axis. Eur J Immunol 19: 301–305

Subject Index

Current Topics in Microbiology and Immunology

Volumes published since 1986 (and still available)

Vol. 129: 1986. 43 figs., VII, 215 pp.
ISBN 3-540-16834-6

Vol. 130: **Koprowski, Hilary; Melchers, Fritz (Ed.):** Peptides as Immunogens. 1986. 21 figs. X, 86 pp. ISBN 3-540-16892-3

Vol. 131: **Doerfler, Walter; Böhm, Petra (Ed.):** The Molecular Biology of Baculoviruses. 1986. 44 figs. VIII, 169 pp. ISBN 3-540-17073-1

Vol. 132: **Melchers, Fritz; Potter, Michael (Ed.):** Mechanisms in B-Cell Neoplasia. Workshop at the National Cancer, Institute, National Institutes of Health, Bethesda, MD, USA, March 24–26, 1986. 1986. 156 figs. XII, 374 pp. ISBN 3-540-17048-0

Vol. 133: **Oldstone, Michael B. (Ed.):** Arenaviruses. Genes, Proteins, and Expression. 1987. 39 figs. VII, 116 pp. ISBN 3-540-17246-7

Vol. 134: **Oldstone, Michael B. (Ed.):** Arenaviruses. Biology and Imminotherapy. 1987. 33 figs. VII, 242 pp. ISBN 3-540-14322-6

Vol. 135: **Paige, Christopher J.; Gisler, Roland H. (Ed.):** Differentiation of B Lymphocytes. 1987. 25 figs. IX, 150 pp. ISBN 3-540-17470-2

Vol. 136: **Hobom, Gerd; Rott, Rudolf (Ed.):** The Molecular Biology of Bacterial Virus Systems. 1988. 20 figs. VII, 90 pp. ISBN 3-540-18513-5

Vol. 137: **Mock, Beverly; Potter, Michael (Ed.):** Genetics of Immunological Diseases. 1988. 88 figs. XI, 335 pp. ISBN 3-540-19253-0

Vol. 138: **Goebel, Werner (Ed.):** Intracellular Bacteria. 1988. 18 figs. IX, 179 pp. ISBN 3-540-50001-4

Vol. 139: **Clarke, Adrienne E.; Wilson, Ian A. (Ed.):** Carbohydrate-Protein Interaction. 1988. 35 figs. IX, 152 pp. ISBN 3-540-19378-2

Vol. 140: **Podack, Eckhard R. (Ed.):** Cytotoxic Effector Mechanisms. 1989. 24 figs. VIII, 126 pp. ISBN 3-540-50057-X

Vol. 141: **Potter, Michael; Melchers, Fritz (Ed.):** Mechanisms in B-Cell Neoplasia 1988. Workshop at the National Cancer Institute, National Institutes of Health, Bethesda, MD, USA, March 23–25, 1988. 1988. 122 figs. XIV, 340 pp. ISBN 3-540-50212-2

Vol. 142: **Schüpach, Jörg:** Human Retrovirology. Facts and Concepts. 1989. 24 figs. 115 pp. ISBN 3-540-50455-9

Vol. 143: **Haase, Ashley T.; Oldstone Michael B. A. (Ed.):** In Situ Hybridization 1989. 22 figs. XII, 90 pp. ISBN 3-540-50761-2

Vol. 144: **Knippers, Rolf; Levine, A. J. (Ed.):** Transforming. Proteins of DNA Tumor Viruses. 1989. 85 figs. XIV, 300 pp. ISBN 3-540-50909-7

Vol. 145: **Oldstone, Michael B. A. (Ed.):** Molecular Mimicry. Cross-Reactivity between Microbes and Host Proteins as a Cause of Autoimmunity. 1989. 28 figs. VII, 141 pp. ISBN 3-540-50929-1

Vol. 146: **Mestecky, Jiri; McGhee, Jerry (Ed.):** New Strategies for Oral Immunization. International Symposium at the University of Alabama at Birmingham and Molecular Engineering Associates, Inc. Birmingham, AL, USA, March 21–22, 1988. 1989. 22 figs. IX, 237 pp. ISBN 3-540-50841-4

Vol. 147: **Vogt, Peter K. (Ed.):** Oncogenes. Selected Reviews. 1989. 8 figs. VII, 172 pp. ISBN 3-540-51050-8

Vol. 148: **Vogt, Peter K. (Ed.):** Oncogenes and Retroviruses. Selected Reviews. 1989. XII, 134 pp. ISBN 3-540-51051-6

Vol. 149: **Shen-Ong, Grace L. C.; Potter, Michael; Copeland, Neal G. (Ed.):** Mechanisms in Myeloid Tumorigenesis. Workshop at the National Cancer Institute, National Institutes of Health, Bethesda, MD, USA, March 22, 1988. 1989. 42 figs. X, 172 pp. ISBN 3-540-50968-2

Vol. 150: **Jann, Klaus; Jann, Barbara (Ed.):** Bacterial Capsules. 1989. 33 figs. XII, 176 pp. ISBN 3-540-51049-4

Vol. 151: **Jann, Klaus; Jann, Barbara (Ed.):** Bacterial Adhesins. 1990. 23 figs. XII, 192 pp. ISBN 3-540-51052-4

Vol. 152: **Bosma, Melvin J.; Phillips, Robert A.; Schuler, Walter (Ed.):** The Scid Mouse. Characterization and Potential Uses. EMBO Workshop held at the Basel Institute for Immunology, Basel, Switzerland, February 20–22, 1989. 1989. 72 figs. XII, 263 pp. ISBN 3-540-51512-7

Vol. 153: **Lambris, John D. (Ed.):** The Third Component of Complement. Chemistry and Biology. 1989. 38 figs. X, 251 pp. ISBN 3-540-51513-5

Vol. 154: **McDougall, James K. (Ed.):** Cytomegaloviruses. 1990. 58 figs. IX, 286 pp. ISBN 3-540-51514-3

Vol. 155: **Kaufmann, Stefan H. E. (Ed.):** T-Cell Paradigms in Parasitic and Bacterial Infections. 1990. 24 figs. IX, 162 pp. ISBN 3-540-51515-1

Vol. 156: **Dyrberg, Thomas (Ed.):** The Role of Viruses and the Immune System in Diabetes Mellitus. 1990. 15 figs. XI, 142 pp. ISBN 3-540-51918-1

Vol. 157: **Swanstrom, Ronald; Vogt, Peter K. (Ed.):** Retroviruses. Strategies of Replication. 1990. 40 figs. XII, 260 pp. ISBN 3-540-51895-9

Vol. 158: **Muzyczka, Nicholas (Ed.):** Viral Expression Vectors. 1992. Approx. 20 figs. Approx. XII, 190 pp. ISBN 3-540-52431-2

Vol. 159: **Gray, David; Sprent, Jonathan (Ed.):** Immunological Memory. 1990. 38 figs. XII, 156 pp. ISBN 3-540-51921-1

Vol. 160: **Oldstone, Michael B. A.; Koprowski, Hilary (Ed.):** Retrovirus Infections of the Nervous System. 1990. 16 figs. XII, 176 pp. ISBN 3-540-51939-4

Vol. 161: **Racaniello, Vincent R. (Ed.):** Picornaviruses. 1990. 12 figs. X, 194 pp. ISBN 3-540-52429-0

Vol. 162: **Roy, Polly; Gorman, Barry M. (Ed.):** Bluetongue Viruses. 1990. 37 figs. X, 200 pp. ISBN 3-540-51922-X

Vol. 163: **Turner, Peter C.; Moyer, Richard W. (Ed.):** Poxviruses. 1990. 23 figs. X, 210 pp. ISBN 3-540-52430-4

Vol. 164: **Bækkeskov, Steinnun; Hansen, Bruno (Ed.):** Human Diabetes. 1990. 9 figs. X, 198 pp. ISBN 3-540-52652-8

Vol. 165: **Bothwell, Mark (Ed.):** Neuronal Growth Factors. 1991. 14 figs. IX, 173 pp. ISBN 3-540-52654-4

Vol. 166: **Potter, Michael; Melchers, Fritz (Ed.):** Mechanisms in B-Cell Neoplasia 1990. 143 figs. XIX, 380 pp. ISBN 3-540-52886-5

Vol. 167: **Kaufmann, Stefan H. E. (Ed.):** Heat Shock Proteins and Immune Response. 1991. 18 figs. IX, 214 pp. ISBN 3-540-52857-1

Vol. 168: **Mason, William S.; Seeger, Christoph (Ed.):** Hepadnaviruses. Molecular Biology and Pathogenesis. 1991. 21 figs. X, 206 pp. ISBN 3-540-53060-6

Vol. 169: **Kolakofsky, Daniel (Ed.):** Bunyaviridae. 1991. 34 figs. X, 256 pp. ISBN 3-540-53061-4

Vol. 170: **Compans, Richard W. (Ed.):** Protein Traffic in Eukaryotic Cells. Selected Reviews. 1991. 14 figs. X, 186 pp. ISBN 3-540-53631-0

Vol. 171: **Kung, Hsing-Jien (Ed.):** Retroviral Insertional Mutagenesis and Oncogene. 1991. 18 figs. X, 179 pp. ISBN 3-540-53857-7

Vol. 172: **Chesebro, Bruce W. (Ed.):** Transmissible Spongiform Encephalopathies. 1991. 48 figs. X, 288 pp. ISBN 3-540-53883-6

Vol. 173: **Pfeffer, Klaus; Heeg, Klaus; Wagner, Hermann; Riethmüller, Gert (Ed.):** Function and Specificity of γ/δ T Cells. 1991. 41 figs. XII, 296 pp. ISBN 3-540-53781-3